PRACTICE ENHANCEMENT

PRACTICE

The Physician's Guide to

ENHANCEMENT

Success in Private Practice

Greg N. Korneluk
President, The Practice Enhancement Institute
Formerly with the American Medical Association

MACMILLAN PUBLISHING COMPANY
NEW YORK

Collier Macmillan Canada, Inc.
TORONTO

Collier Macmillan Publishers
LONDON

Macmillan Publishing Company
866 Third Avenue, New York, New York 10022

Collier Macmillan Canada, Inc.

Library of Congress Cataloging in Publication Data

Korneluk, Greg N.
  Practice enhancement.

  Includes index.
    1. Medicine—Practice.   2. Ambulatory medical care—
Marketing.   3. Physician and patient.   I. Title.
[DNLM: 1. Marketing of Health Services.   2. Private
Practice—economics.   3. Private Practice—
organization & administration.   W 89 K84p]
R728.K67   1985   610'.68   84–21392
ISBN 0–02–362930–4

Printing: 2 3 4 5 6 7 8   Year: 6 7 8 9 0 1 2 3

To Pat, Keith & Kristen

Preface

————————————————————————●

Competition has invaded the practice of medicine. Once the secure domain of private practitioners, the provision of health care has become big business. With that development, physicians now face some unprecedented and disconcerting challenges, and the traditional physician-patient relationship is undergoing change.

Some sources of competition are the health maintenance organizations, freestanding clinic chains, satellites of group practices which, armed with sophisticated marketing, advertising, and promotional strategies, are competing aggressively for patients. Another problem is the trend toward an oversupply of physicians. Clearly these and other forces at work in our society today require physicians in private practice to become skilled managers—even more, skilled marketers—as well as skilled clinicians.

This book takes a penetrating look at these issues and charts a strategy for survival, growth, and success of the private practice—whether it is an individual practice, partnership, or larger group practice. *Practice Enhancement* takes a "how to" approach, offering concrete solutions to specific problems facing the practitioner. At the heart of the challenge is the patient-physician relationship. This book offers new ideas for developing and nurturing that relationship, for improving patient satisfaction, physician and staff efficiency and satisfaction, and the profitability of the practice.

Acknowledgments

———————————————————————●

Hundreds of physicians in private practices have profoundly influenced the content of these pages. Most of the ideas presented in this book have been learned during ten years of grappling with the day-to-day problems faced by physicians struggling to provide quality care in a changing society.

Special thanks must go to the many physicians with whom I have worked on a consulting basis and who have provided me with the wealth of experiences that have made this book possible. Their numerous ideas, problems, and practices inspired this effort.

The American Medical Association, my former employer, greatly contributed to the formulation of many of my ideas on quality care and the delivery of medical services by private practitioners.

Many of the ideas in this book have been influenced by the following speciality societies and health care organizations: the Canadian Medical Asssociation, the American Hospital Association, the American Society of Internal Medicine, the American Academy of Family Practice, the American Academy of Ophthalmology, the American College of Radiology, the American Academy of Pediatrics, the American Society of Plastic and Reconstructive Surgeons, and the American College of Surgeons.

I would also like to thank the many excellent journals on practice management that published my articles, and allowed me to develop more fully my ideas on practice enhancement—most notably, the magazines *Medical Economics, Physicians Management,* and *Canadian Doctor,* as well as the *Wall Street Journal.*

Contents

The Author

—————————————————————————————●

Greg Korneluk is an internationally recognized consultant, lecturer, and writer on successful practice Enhancement.

Formerly with the American Medical Association, he has traveled extensively, lecturing to and consulting with physicians, dentists, and administrators.

He has been profiled in the *Wall Street Journal,* the *New York Times,* and *Chicago Tribune,* and has written many articles on practice enhancement that have appeared in *Medical Economics, Physicians Management, American Medical Association News, Canadian Medical Association Journal,* and many other Canadian and American journals. In addition, he has appeared on programs sponsored by the American Medical Association, the Canadian Medical Association, the American College of Radiology, the American Academy of Pediatrics, the American Society of Plastic and Reconstructive Surgeons, the American Society of Abdominal Surgeons, the American Dental Association, and many others.

A practice productivity specialist, he also provides consulting services in medical marketing, doctor time management, practice efficiency, personal financial planning, accounting, personnel administration, associate relations, group practice organization, computerization, patient management, and other related health services areas. His clients include many successful physicians in individual partnership and group practices as well as a number of major hospitals, universities, medical societies, and health care corporations.

Introduction

The traditional practice of medicine is undergoing a metamorphosis in the way services are delivered. Three key elements involved in this change include competition caused by physician oversupply, the rising cost of health care services, and the consumer health movement. To survive and prosper in this turbulent time, physicians will continue to face new challenges brought about by the combination of these factors.

This book offers a system for practice success that addresses these issues and focuses on practice survival in a competitive era as its central emphasis. This process, which I term practice enhancement, takes the best of the traditional practice management model and blends it with new marketing methods into a system that assists the quality conscious physician to meet the new competition.

As medicine matures and moves from a "cottage industry"—one where patient service is delivered by many individual small practices—to one that is dominated by group and corporate enterprises, individual private practitioners will be threatened by new forms of competition. We have already witnessed the inroads into traditional patient bases by health maintenance organizations and preferred provider organizations, which offer discounts and a new philosophy of practice. Satellite facilities and innovative corporate-sponsored facilities will also continue to erode patient bases. Practice enhancement can help you meet the challenges posed by these new forms of services.

Physician oversupply will continue at least until the year 2000, while demand for medical service will diminish during this period, according to Graduate Medical Education National Advisory Committee (GMENAC) to the Department of Health and Human Services. This physician oversupply will send ripples throughout the health care community and affect virtually every physician's practice. By enhancing your practice, you will better withstand the impact of change and minimize your personal risk.

The trend of continually rising health care costs has led to pressure from government, business, unions, and consumers for ways to contain costs. As momentum grows and as patients become more open to alternative forms of health care, physicians will require systems to control costs. An effective practice enhancement method incorporates cost containment as a central concept to maintain a viable practice.

As patient attitudes begin to change from the traditional model in which the patient accepted the judgments of trained professionals and institutions as gospel to one that is more questioning, more pressure will be exerted on the medical profession. The consumer movement, which gained momentum in the 1960s and 1970s and is now reaching a peak, has readied the ultimate consumer of health services to accept and even influence changes in the health care system. Practice enhancement helps address the new patient attitudes within a workable methodology.

As more and more physicians serve fewer and fewer patients, as more pressure is placed on containing costs, and as patients become consumer advocates, tremendous change will be felt throughout the health care community; the successful practitioners will have to make fundamental changes in their practices to survive. Careful guidelines, which can be provided by a practice enhancement system, will help the quality-oriented physician pinpoint necessary practice changes that can ensure a desirable practice outcome.

Competition

The oversupply of physicians has contributed to the competitive climate more than has any other variable. In addition to the increased competition between private practitioners vying for patients, new forms of health services also deflect patients from the traditional approach to medical care. These alternative forms of care include corporations that deliver medical care with establishments that resemble business franchises, medical centers set up for the convenience of the patient, strengthened health maintenance organizations (HMOs) in urban areas, and preferred provider organizations (PPOs). Because health care is now viewed on Wall Street as a growth business, new financial capital is being infused into this field.

As a result of corporate involvement and other financing, large expensive facilities are being established to offer fast, convenient, and reasonably priced medical services to patients. There is no doubt that the impact of these new establishments on the delivery of primary and secondary care services in health care will be enormous. Patients will be exposed to new and different approaches and will begin to expect a similar level of service from all physicians.

Hospitals, seeing that their referrals are threatened by the changing patterns established by the competing forces, are looking at ways to strengthen their referral base. Joint venture arrangements between hospitals and medical staffs may establish free-standing satellite facilities, and hospitals can provide physicians with sound management advice. However, the goal of the hospitals is to protect their own survival and in many cases this is in conflict with loyal medical practitioners. Still, these joint venture arrangements will become more necessary as a means of meeting increased competition.

Finally, physicians face a new level of competition from a group they nurtured when doctors were scarce—the physician assistants and other paramedicals, including independent nurse practitioners, nutritionists, nurse midwives, physiotherapists, and others. In addition, chiropractors, podiatrists, optometrists, dentists, and pharmacists are beginning to encroach into areas that were once the domain of physicians.

Cost Control

As the finance departments of corporations begin to develop incentives for employees to cut health costs and look for alternative forms of care, further pressure will be exerted on the traditional systems of delivering care. Legislation and the efforts of the Federal Trade Commission will also continue to encourage competition as a method of driving prices down. The Justice Department and the FTC have aggressively pursued any organized groups that have attempted to restrain trade by barring marketing and advertising as unethical; this has also stimulated the competitive climate.

As government continues to refine the system of prospective payment for medical services called diagnostic related groups (DRGs), it will continue the pressure for reducing cost within the system. As a result, we will see more pressure from businesses who pay health care costs along with government to find alternative methods of reducing costs and stimulating competition. In a number of corporations, health care services represent the single largest expense after direct labor costs. The automobile industry has reported that health care is close to 5 percent of the total cost of some cars. Since businesses pay the health care premium, it is only appropriate that they seek methods to decrease cost for health care. Some cost control methods include coalitions of businessmen to study the problem and the use of comparison shopping for medical care.

Role of the Patient

Patients—the focus of the health care system—are undergoing some fundamental changes in their attitudes about their health, as shown by the growth of the self-care movement. Self-help books and health-oriented magazines are currently bringing great success to their publishers. Also, patients can now purchase over-the-counter kits for a number of medical tests that they could previously only get from their doctors. For example, patients can perform pregnancy tests, throat cultures, urine tests, and bowel cancer screening, as well as monitor their blood pressure and pulse, just to name a few. This trend toward increased self-care seems likely to continue to grow. Patients have also shown greater sophistication in their knowledge of medicine, possibly as a result of greater scientific and technological awareness in this growingly computerized society.

Patients are also becoming more informed consumers and are shopping for doctors; as they become more demanding, they force physicians to reevaluate their service. Patient attitudes regarding their physician and health care have been traditionally slow to change. Most patients still view their health care as something that should be decided by the experts. However, as books and other media expose patients to new thinking and new ways of delivering care, they are becoming more open to change.

Application of the Practice Enhancement System

In the changing, competitive environment, it is necessary to reassess the traditional practice management model, which typically focuses on maintaining practice costs and maximizing efficiency; our emphasis should shift from that model to incorporate aspects of the marketing model, which has valuable techniques to offer. The approach that I call practice enhancement represents a careful blending of the best of traditional methods with contemporary marketing ideas.

Practice enhancement focuses on the critical issues that surround practice growth. The central theme of practice enhancement is that your patients are primary (or, as they say in the business world, "the customer is king"). Successful practitioners have always put patient needs, wants, and expectations first, above practice management systems and procedures and personal satisfaction. The most successful practices of the future will specifically focus on patient wants and perceptions as the primary emphasis for a satisfying and prosperous practice.

Practice Management Aspects

Practice enhancement takes the traditional practice management thinking regarding systems such as collections, telephone management, and appointment scheduling and emphasizes patient satisfaction as the reason for efficiency and good service. For example, in this system, collection systems are tailored to match patient attitudes regarding financial arrangements; thus, more effort will be placed on projecting positive healthy approaches to money rather than the end result of getting money into the bank.

With practice enhancement, every management system in your practice should be reviewed from the perspective of the patient to ensure that it is patient centered and maximizes satisfaction. In the past, if a practice system alienated a patient and he or she never came back, there was always another patient ready and willing to fill that spot. Because this is no longer true, physicians will have to be careful in how the systems are structured to ensure patient satisfaction.

Use of Marketing Model

Practice enhancement also incorporates many positive ideas from the marketing model and applies them to your practice. It is my opinion that if you expect to be a successful practitioner in the 1980s and 1990s, you must incorporate marketing techniques into your personal practice enhancement program. These marketing ideas relate more to what I call your augmented service, which represents areas in which patients normally evaluate their satisfaction with their doctor, rather than to your main service—the actual care that you deliver. Your personal style, the pleasantness of your staff, the convenience of your location, your practice policies, and your facilities are the most important aspects of your augmented service, and these features constitute the central focus of this book.

Throughout the book I will attempt to show you how to apply the marketing concept to your practice. Marketing techniques can give you a competitive edge by helping you keep your patients happy. Clearly, the forces that work in the marketplace require that you become both an expert manager and a skilled practitioner—some say that as a physician of the future you must also be a talented marketer to be successful.

This book takes a penetrating look at the growth, expansion, and survival of private medicine. It provides new ideas to enhance your practice, help improve patient satisfaction, physician and staff efficiency, and the profitability of private practice and offers concrete solutions to problems currently facing the medical profession.

Audience for This Book

The book is written specifically for those physicians (especially those in private practice) and organizations who want to maintain the competitive edge in medical practice. I have tried to incorporate specific suggestions that will make it possible to stay one step ahead of the competition. This approach demands that we take a positive attitude about the changes that we are about to encounter.

Physicians going into practice for the first time will find this book useful in the development of a practice management philosophy; some specific systems and procedures that are described may be especially successful if they are incorporated at the beginning of a practice.

Independent physicians and members of group practices considering adding a partner or opening satellite facilities will find a number of the concepts in this book useful in its overall approach to the development of the practice.

Requirements for a Successful Practice

This book is organized around the five critical building blocks to a comprehensive patient-centered practice: (1) patient orientation, (2) staff members, (3) practice procedures, (4) attitude and leadership of the physician, and (5) the relationship of the physician to his or her colleagues.

Patient Orientation

You must understand the changing attitudes of today's patient toward medicine. The wants and needs of the patient (or customer) are central to the delivery of your service. It is important to understand how patients think, how they view your practice, how they are motivated, and most specifically, how to satisfy them. The chapters in the first section (Your Patients) deal with patient orientation and patient management issues.

To establish a patient orientation, you need to understand the marketing process, the language of marketing, and the way that competition affects your practice. The method for accomplishing this is to conduct a marketing audit of your practice, to reexamine a number of your long-held attitudes, and to evaluate the patient handling systems in your practice. You will have to pay closer attention to pricing strategies and to your location, and it is also important to develop new systems in your practice, such as patient retention programs, patient accounting, monitoring feedback from your patients, low-key promotional programs, and other methods for improving your patients' satisfaction.

Staff Members

The people on your staff are the true ambassadors of your practice. You must understand and be able to discern what type of individual you should hire, how to recruit them, how to train them, and how to keep them. You should try to employ staff members who genuinely care about patients and who can take an interest in the growth of your practice. You will need to examine organizational techniques for the development of an effective organization, to develop patient-centered job descriptions, to evaluate your staff's performance, and to implement personnel policies that make sense. These topics are covered in more detail in the second section (Your Staff).

Practice Procedures

Your methods for booking appointments, collecting from patients, and filing records greatly affect the level of service you provide. Obviously, a successful practice has to have very tight procedures in order to deliver the high level of service expected by the consumer-oriented patient. Moreover, the emphasis on cost control within these systems will be critical. The chapters in the third section (Your Practice) deal with specific systems and procedures needed to deliver your service effectively.

To improve your practice systems and procedures, not only do you need to look at patient satisfaction, but you must also consider ways of increasing your productivity without sacrificing patient service to ensure your competitive viability from a standpoint of cost efficiency. As a result, you should reevaluate your financial systems, appointment scheduling systems, telephone handling techniques, medical records management, facilities planning, and financial management. Only through implementing efficient procedures that are patient oriented will your practice continue to be strong.

Attitude and Leadership of the Physician

The physician's attitude and leadership are the most important variables contributing to patient satisfaction and to the growth and success of the practice. The final section of this book will cover the attitudes and skills you must develop in order to increase the growth of your practice. It is essential that you understand your patients' needs and expectations in order to keep your "customers" satisfied.

Relationship of Physicians with Colleagues

The chapters in the last section of this book discuss the ways that you deal with your colleagues. If you are in a referral practice relations with colleagues are especially important. You need to understand the implications of your personal style, your telephone technique, and the way that you delegate responsibility in your practice. Referrals will become increasingly important as competition grows. As your practice expands, you may wish to address the issue of choosing a partner or of determining the true value of your practice. Since a medical practice is becoming more of a business, business techniques will be critical to your survival.

To compete effectively in today's medical community you must understand the expectations that your patients have derived from dealing with other service firms. In evaluating service, consumers weigh the cost, convenience, and quality of their purchases. The time has now come when they are evaluating your medical service by the same criteria.

Throughout the book, I will share specific examples of how medical practices have responded to the competitive challenge, suggest guidelines for some specific changes necessary in your practice, and give examples of forms that I have found successful in various practices that I have worked with.

I believe that private practice, as a primary mechanism for the delivery of patient care, will survive competitive challenges because of its ability to adapt quickly. It was private enterprise that helped our health care system become the best in the world; the system will continue to deliver quality patient-oriented services for many years to come if we go back to the roots of the success—namely, keeping the patient satisfied.

Your Patients

Your patients are the most valuable assets in your practice. To develop a thriving and successful medical practice, you need to pay close attention to four important variables—knowing your patients, attracting them, satisfying them, and keeping them.

Competition and marketing directly affect your patients. Chapter 1 will help you understand the marketing process and how it can be utilized as a useful tool in your practice enhancement program. The new language (or jargon) of marketing will be discussed in Chapter 2.

Knowing your patients begins with a comprehensive analysis of your practice, as is spelled out in detail in Chapter 3, which describes how to conduct a marketing audit of your practice (a specific method that allows you to assess your situation in an organized way). Close attention should be given to understanding the special needs of your patients as health services purchasers.

Viewing your patients as purchasers of health services requires a new perspective on the old practice management model. Chapter 4 will help you look at how you set your fee and how you price your services from your patients' standpoint.

Chapter 5 looks at ways of assessing a location, which will be important to physicians who wish to reevaluate their current location or who are looking at new locations for a practice or for a satellite facility. Location will become a more crucial variable to practice growth as competition increases.

Most practices grow through word-of-mouth promotion, which can be augmented by marketing methods. As described in Chapter 6, a patient retention program can help you decrease patient attrition.

Critical to practice growth is the understanding of patient satisfaction with your service. As your reputation for being a competent and courteous physician increases, you will steadily add to your patient roster. If all the critical elements of the practice management mix are well integrated into a quality service, these satisfied patients will refer still others to your practice. Chapter 7 will help you manage patient growth through patient accounting.

By keeping in touch with your patients through surveys and with a patient retention program, you will stay one step ahead of your competition. Chapter 8 discusses how you can pay close attention to your patients' satisfaction with your location and to any specific problems your patients might have with your practice. That chapter gives examples of specific methods for obtaining feedback from your patients about their attitudes to your practice.

Promotional techniques can also be used for practice expansion;

however, you should never be more aggressive that you have to be. Chapter 9 specifically addresses what promotion can work for you.

You are more likely to keep your patients if you understand their expectations of your practice. Patients come to you because of your reputation as a quality practitioner, but they probably stay with you because of your augmented service—those issues that relate to appointment scheduling, location, and staff courtesy—rather than the actual medical care. Chapter 10 looks at patient satisfaction and what you should do in considering this important issue.

The delicate balance between knowing your patients, attracting them, satisfying them, and keeping them can be maintained by understanding and using the marketing concept and applying it to your practice. Patient satisfaction is an elusive issue. If you are sensitive to the changing values of your patients, your patients will be happier and will refer you to others whom it will be a pleasure for you to serve. The marketing process can help ensure your success when used as part of an overall well-thought-out practice enhancement program.

Chapter 1

Competition and Marketing Do Affect Your Practice

When we think of marketing, we have many negative images and emotions—the flimflam man selling his wares, Madison Avenue hype, physicians' names on bulletin boards in lights, and an overall tainted association with hucksterism. Yet, as we examine more closely the concepts and ideas behind marketing, which is a recognized discipline in the most prestigious business schools, we will see how it can become a constructive tool to build the success of your practice and maximize patient compliance and satisfaction. Whether you like it, or (most probably) not, marketing has come to medicine and it is here to stay.

Today, it is almost becoming a prerequisite to use marketing techniques just to maintain the status quo. Many successful group practices and practitioners have been using marketing techniques for years to build practices, improve patient compliance, and maximize patient satisfaction. The more you examine the marketing idea, the more you will begin to understand why renowned medical clinics are writing marketing plans and why hospitals are appointing specialists to implement comprehensive strategic marketing plans. Why? Because it gets results.

What is Marketing?

I define marketing (when applied to a medical practice) as a dynamic system of coordinated activities centering on the interchanges between patients and the practice, whose objective is to improve patient well-being, compliance, and satisfaction, in a cost-effective manner, for the benefit of the patient and the medical practice. A less formal explanation is that marketing involves understanding your patients' needs and desires, and organizing your practice to ensure that the level of services delivered meets these expectations.

The marketing concept is a working model that can help you organize your decisions regarding practice planning, setting fees, promoting your practice, and delivering your services to your patients to ensure practice growth and patient happiness. It takes into account all those critical activities that influence your patients' perception of your practice and helps you create a balance that helps ensure your success.

It is important to understand that marketing is a dynamic continuum of activities, ranging from very passive and conservative strategies to very aggressive ones. For example, listing your address and phone number in the telephone book is marketing. Taking out a quarter-page advertisement in the yellow pages is merely a more aggressive version of the same process. Although both activities represent forms of marketing, it is the more flamboyant approach of taking the quarter-page advertisement or purchasing a paid advertisement in an airline journal that is most distasteful to private practitioners. However as competition increases, practitioners will be forced to become more aggressive with their promotional approaches to maintain their visibility.

The Concept of Augmented Service Versus Core Service

In developing your practice enhancement program you should focus on the augmented services that facilitate the delivery of medical care—appointment booking, telephone answering, your patient orientation, your facility, the pleasantness of your staff, the ease of making appointments, and so on. (The care you deliver to your patients is your core service.) Most patients do not judge their physicians by the delivery of the basic medical care. Rather, they put more emphasis in judging the augmented services, because the actual care is often too complex or too elusive for them to comprehend. If well managed, augmented services can enhance your core service by positively influencing your patients. (Your core service, however, does need to be carefully assessed in the development of your marketing program; the next chapter will discuss the need for a quantitative and qualitative understanding of your core service as obtained by making a marketing audit.)

It is my contention that medical practices, more than any other service businesses, have become attuned to the wants and needs of patients. Physicians acting in response to their patients wishes are using marketing concepts. A marketing-oriented practice is a continually changing entity. As patients' needs change and competition among practices for patients increases, more aggressive contemporary creative approaches will have to be taken by practitioners in order to survive.

Uses of Marketing Approaches

The consumerism that has come to medicine is reflected in patients who are taking more interest in their medical care and becoming active participants in that care. One result of the consumerism patients display is increased litigation; the fear of malpractice suits is valid. There have even been successful suits in small claims courts in New Jersey and Oregon by patients complaining of long waits in reception rooms. We will see more of this aggressive behavior as we move into the future, but a marketing framework will help us minimize the problem. Marketing concepts help us understand how the consumer health movement affects patients and in turn how to motivate and work with patients for their benefit and the benefit of the practice.

The negative emotional responses that many doctors have to marketing relate to the fact that there are many misconceptions about it. Marketing is not advertising, selling, or public relations. Nor is it hucksterism used to create unnecessary demand for medical services; rather, it is a recognized, legitimate management function in profit-making and nonprofit businesses and medical practices. Just as we have a planned approach to long-term patient management, we can use marketing techniques as part of our practice enhancement program to facilitate long-term practice success.

Marketing focuses on the needs of your patients, while selling focuses on the needs of the physician or provider. Typically, in discussions revolving around marketing by physicians, it is always discussed in the same context as selling, advertising, or promotion. This is only a small part of the overall concept and should be recognized as such.

How Marketing Techniques Can Work For You

The theory, principles, techniques, and philosophies of marketing are the same whether you are in solo practice, in partnership practice, in a small group, or part of a large practice. The following are some specific tips to help you in assessing marketing opportunities in your area:

1. Pay very close attention to patient complaints about medical services in your region, and make sure they are not prevalent in your own practice.
2. Assign someone on your staff to treat every patient complaint in your practice as a number one priority. Give this staff member the title Patient Relations Coordinator.
3. Understand population shifts in your area and the spending habits of the residents. Go to your library and Chamber of Commerce to examine federal census and demographic studies.
4. Look to see what physicians in large and successful practices are doing. Perhaps they are filling a special need that you could fill too. For example, are they offering evening hours, free blood-pressure clinics, or patient-education classes?
5. Look for practices with new and innovative ideas and apply these to your practice.
6. Survey your patients for their feedback on your practice procedures.

These are just few specific programs and ideas that should be integrated in a marketing plan for your practice. Later in the book we will deal specifically with how to conduct a medical practice audit in the development of this plan.

Some Applications of Marketing Conccepts

Relocation of a Practice

Location analysis and demographic shifts are critical in the marketing process as it applies to medical practices. One example of this situation involves a pediatrician in a midwestern town who found that his patient load had been declining over a period of six years. Fortunately, his wife was studying geography at a local university and decided to focus her demographics project on the choice of a better location for his practice. She applied demographic statistics to urban geography, and her understanding of market research methodology enabled her to make this project a success.

After conducting some extensive market research, she found that her husband had located in an area where the population under 18 was declining rapidly. A study of the region indicated that the new families with young children were locating in a different section of town. On the basis of this information, the pediatrician relocated his practice in an area where the population of children was increasing, and he is now doing well.

As you can see, marketing encompasses many different disciplines. With a little analysis and understanding of patient demographic shifts, the marketing process was brought to bear for the successful growth and development of this pediatrician's practice.

Changing Patient Mix

A Boston physician specializing in obstetrics and gynecology found that 75 percent of his practice was primary care. His marketing objective was to increase the percentage of gynecological surgery patients. The overriding problem was that he was then working at full capacity, which made any change difficult.

The first step in restructuring his practice was to develop a patient information booklet detailing his new policy of seeing only patients with emergencies and those who needed surgery. He also formulated a policy of seeing only patients who were referred by another physician, and communicated this via the information booklet. In addition, he designed a number of questions to allow his assistants to screen patients before accepting them into his practice (he had previously not done any screening). The questions were designed to ascertain beforehand whether the patient had complicated problems that required his attention. New patients needing primary care were not accepted.

Over a period of three years, his patient mix changed to meet his goal of reducing his primary care load to 30 percent. This objective was achieved through natural patient attrition, consistent patient education (via the telephone by his assistants, as well as through patient information booklets sent in the mail), and reinforcement by the physician. In some situations where patients had been with the doctor for more than 15 years, the physician personally sent letters to these patients saying that he was available for their surgery and specifically recommending two other doctors in town that he felt could meet their primary care requirements. The 30 percent of patients who needed primary care were mainly those for whom surgery was indicated but who had not yet made up their minds to proceed.

As you can see, the successful marketing program begins by identifying the problem. In this case, the surgeon wanted to change the mix of his patients. The next step was to structure the practice promotion, which included writing a patient information booklet detailing the policy and developing a sales program with the staff and physician describing the new policy to already established patients. The combination of promotion and sales helped this practitioner achieve his marketing objective.

Mobile Care Center

A New Jersey psychiatric group learned that their older patient population found it hard getting to their facility. As a solution, the doctors set up a mental health center on wheels, which provided (on an informal basis) the services of a mental health nurse, counselor-driver, and social worker. In addition to mental health counseling, the service provided testing for hypertension, audiometric screening, and information and referral services for the elderly. The program increased awareness of the group's services and the mobile center proved to be a valuable resource to the patient population.

As you are beginning to see, marketing can be a very useful discipline that can benefit your patients and your practice. When coupled with good practice management systems it can become a philosophy and a tool that can be used to improve patient satisfaction and practice profitability. Use it prudently. With it you will be able to meet the competitive challenges and succeed in building a thriving practice.

●

Chapter 2

The New Language of Marketing

Marketing is a management discipline with its own special language and jargon. To understand marketing (and keep the edge on the competition), we must learn its language. The following are a number of marketing words that I have defined in the context of a medical practice.

Ability-to-Pay Pricing. Pricing on the basis of a patient's ability to pay. For example, in many practices Medicare and Medicaid patients pay less for the same quality of care than private patients.

Account Executive. The person at the advertising agency who is responsible for coordinating your advertising program; he or she is your liaison between you and the creative people at the advertising agency, and is ultimately responsible for the positive execution of your advertising program.

Advertising. A controlled method of communicating the viewpoint of your practice to patients. Typically, you pay for your message, control its content, and select the media—for example, yellow pages, radio, direct mail, television, and billboards.

Augmented Service. As compared to your *core service,* this pertains to the intangible aspects of your practice by which patients judge your practice quality. Augmented services include such things as your personal style, the pleasantness of your staff, the ease of parking, seeing patients on time, the atmosphere of your facility, your patient information material, overall image, and so on.

Base Price and Extras. The patient is charged a base price for the office visit, and specific services performed—for example, laboratory tests, x-ray studies, suture removals, and so on—are added to the bill.

Box Advertisement. An advertisement (typically in a newspaper) that is run with a solid border outside of the regular column. A premium is usually charged for this format. While normally used for formal announcements (such as the addition of a new partner to your practice), creative copy can also be included in the box.

Brand Identification. A word, slogan, or logo that identifies a specific service or group of services with a particular practice. An example would be the use of the name "Exec-u-physical" to describe the annual physical offered by an executive health center.

Channels of Distribution. The transfer point where medical services are delivered to patients. Some creative channels of distribution include department store clinics, practices in shopping malls, services delivered by doctors using mobile vans, and house call services.

Closed-Door Membership Practice. A type of practice in which new patients must enroll to use its services; they usually pay an initiation fee or annual dues to the practice. These practices typically provide a membership card, newsletter, patient education classes, and other amenities not usually found in private practices.

Competitive Pricing. A method of determining the charges on the basis of what other physicians in the area are charging for a particular procedure. This assumes that patients are price sensitive.

Consumer Analysis. Usually part of the market research function that identifies specific patient characteristics. In the analysis you will determine such items as their average age, sex, outlook on medical practice, lifestyles, and so on. The consumer analysis will help you develop a patient profile that helps you in developing your marketing plan.

Controlled Circulation. Magazines or newspapers control circulation by carefully screening the readers into specific demographic groups in an area. Local newspapers might, for example, cater to a specific suburban area guaranteeing you exposure in your advertising program to a selected geographic location. Other magazines might be aimed specifically at people interested in health, thus exposing your message to a health-centered readership. Careful consideration should be given to controlled circulation publications in your advertising program to maximize its effects.

Cooperative Advertising. Advertising jointly sponsored by several physicians or group practices. Since costs are shared, co-op ads generally promote the image of the profession and its services, rather than any individual practice.

Core Service. The mainstream medical care and patient services provided by traditional physicians to their patients—that is, the actual hands-on care by physician and staff to improve the health of their patient. Most patients do not possess enough medical training to evaluate the quality of your core service, and will pay more attention to your *augmented service.*

Cost Pricing. Pricing based on the actual cost of the service delivered (physician's time, supplies used, overhead, allocation, profit, etc.). This method is in direct contrast to Competitive Pricing which ignores unit costs and uses as its criterion what other practitioners in the area are charging.

Creative Strategy. The practice position paper that directs your final promotion. One example of a creative strategy would be to project your medical practice as one that is highly conservative, professional, competent, and qualified. This strategy would influence how the graphics and typeface in the advertisements looked, the final places the advertisements would run, and how ideas will be translated into the final promotion.

Direct Mail. A promotional mailing to prospective patients that can be used for practice building. It may constitute part of your advertising program. Mailings can be first class, bulk mail, or part of a community package where your advertising piece is one of many.

Discount Medical Centers. Medical practitioners or groups charging lower fees while providing a lower level of augmented service to the patient.

Exurbia. Areas beyond suburbs but still accessible to major city services—more patients are moving into these areas.

Fixed Pricing. Another form of pricing used mainly by health maintenance organizations (HMOs). In this type of pricing, an actuarial calculation is taken of what the cost would be to deliver medical care on a long-term basis, and the patients are quoted a fixed monthly price, regardless of whether they receive the required treatment or not.

Loss Leader. A service delivered at or below cost to bring patients into the practice—for example, the $5 checkup in dentistry, or free health screenings to uncover other major problems that need to be treated. A newer loss leader in medical practice is the free get-acquainted visit for new patients.

Market Penetration. This is your practice's percentage of patients from a specific market. Market penetration is usually discussed in the context of *Market Share*; namely, what percentage of a specific patient group is being serviced by your practice.

Market Research. An organized analysis of information—typically patient and demographic data, on which to base your practice management or marketing plans. The purpose of market research is to isolate specific patient characteristics so that you can respond appropriately. Market research helps you determine the best ways to deliver your services and your message.

Market Segmentation. An analytical approach used to define the demographic characteristics of a patient population. The end result will be some clearly identifiable targets for a marketing program.

Market Share. A mathematical calculation that determines precisely what portion of a particular patient type is under your care. If you are drawing patients from a 40-mile radius, the estimated number of diabetics in your area is 1,000, and your practice has 100 diabetics, then you have 10-percent market share.

Media Mix. Planning the coordination of advertising and promotion—for example, newspaper, radio, television—to present a message. When laying out a promotional budget, you must decide how much you will spend on advertising, public relations, and so on. The final mix of promotional ingredients is your media mix.

Metromarket. Central city plus suburban areas from which a clinic or practitioner may draw patients.

Positioning Strategy. The steps you take to position your practice in the patient's mind as specializing in a particular area. A good example of a positioning strategy would be an executive health clinic. Even though the clinic will see patients who are not executives, the clinic in an affluent suburb positions its medical services for executives in the nearby corporate head offices. Promotion, scheduling, and service caters to busy executives perceiving the need for special services. Positioning strategy always takes into account the position of the market leader and competition.

Practice Clusters. A group of practices located in a geographical area sharing the cost of advertising, centralized purchasing, and staffing, to provide a profitable operation for the group. This is the current strategy for many free-standing urgent care centers.

Profit Squeeze. Generally caused by severe price competition or by increased costs (for example, a 78 percent unexpected increase in malpractice insurance cost in New York State) that cannot be passed directly on to the patient in its entirety in a particular year. As price becomes more of a marketing issue, cost containment will be critical to effective marketing and minimizing profit squeezes.

Public Relations (PR). An indirect method of promoting the positive achievements or viewpoints of your practice. Public relations tends to be news-oriented, uses the traditional media, and is generally free; it takes the form of news releases, statements to the media, public speaking, appearing on talk shows, and writing featured articles. One disadvantage is that the practice does not have control over the final message.

Selling. The objective of selling in a medical practice is to achieve patient compliance. Whether a patient is trying to quit smoking, lose weight, or cope with a particularly difficult method of treatment, he needs to be motivated. The effective medical practice is able to make the patient see all the benefits of complying with the best course of action.

Target Marketing. Directing your efforts to penetrate a specific segment of the available market. A family practice resident was very specific about the patient mix he wanted in his practice. He wanted a good combination of geriatric patients, children, and adults. He targeted his practice on an ethnic area where three generations of the same families lived close to each other. By targeting his market and then doing a socioeconomic demographic analysis, he began to develop the practice mix of his choice.

Test Market. Rather than fully implement a new service or program (for example, asking for payment at the time of service) try it out on a limited basis to gauge patient reaction. If the response is positive, then implement the program. If poor, do not proceed. Many new services or ideas never make it through the test market phase.

Value Pricing. Pricing based on the relative task and complexity of a procedure performed. This method of pricing is used by many surgeons and subspecialty areas, especially for new procedures.

Visual Merchandising. A retail concept that considers the point-of-sale merchandising of your medical practice. It involves dressing your window with a medical theme and developing displays within your reception area and outside of your practice to attract patients. As medical practices begin to open in shopping malls and in highly visible locations, visual merchandising will become more important in drawing patients. As an example, one general practitioner opened a clinic that offered free blood pressure testing. When a sign was posted in the window, the number of patients coming in to take up the offer increased. The sign was an example of good visual merchandising.

As you can see, there is a lot more to marketing than advertising, selling, or public relations. Marketing is a discipline, and by understanding the new language of marketing you will be better equipped to meet the competitive challenge.

●

Chapter 3

How To Conduct a Medical Practice Market Audit

A comprehensive assessment of the strengths and weaknesses of your practice represents a good way to start implementing a practice enhancement program that will help you meet the challenges of the next decade. Your objective should be to develop a plan that anticipates future challenges, keeps your practice growing, and is patient-centered. The process of committing your plan to paper is an excellent way to crystallize your thoughts about your practice. The audit findings are another way of staying one step ahead of the advancing competition.

When first seeing a new patient, the physician takes a comprehensive history and physical before making a diagnosis and choosing a course of treatment. In the business side of practice, the same type of initial evaluation—called a marketing audit—involves an objective assessment of where you've been, where you are now, and where you can go; it also assesses the key areas of practice development that will greatly influence your long-term success.

Assess Your Practice Trade Area

To develop a usable plan, you must first determine what your practice trade area is. This concept, borrowed from retailing, basically states that

80 percent of your patients come from a specific drawing area. When you determine the demographic characteristics of your patients, you will be able to begin to compile statistics about your trade area and complete the rest of the audit.

The specific statistical information that you will need to complete the market audit can be obtained from the most recent census data or from firms specializing in market research. Most companies performing such research can get you a complete population breakdown within specific zip codes or census tracks. All you need to do is send them the zip codes that your patients are living in and they will return to you a number of statistics that will help you assess your trade area. A comparison of demographic characteristics of your patient population with the regional statistics shows you how your practice might deviate from the norm.

In addition to knowing where your patients live, you should try to have an idea of why patients from different regions come to you. Other demographic characteristics of your patients include income, age, sex, family size, and occupation; it is also useful to know where they spend their money. Much of the necessary information can be obtained from your patient records. Places of residence can be indicated by push pins placed in a large map, which can be purchased from a city or county planning office. The pins can be color coded to differentiate residences by age or income groupings. You might, for example, decide that you want to see where families are living compared with where single adults—families could be given red pins and single adults yellow ones. Also, you might want to differentiate between men, women, and children with specific colored pins.

Outlined in the following are the key topics that need to be considered when defining your practice trade area.

1. Identify the boundaries within which 80 percent of your patients live.
2. Define the boundaries within which 80 percent of the last 20 percent of your patients live.
3. Identify all of the key groups (or segments) of patients that make up your practice specialty (in terms of age, sex, attitudes, occupation, and any other relevant categories).
4. Try to establish how each identified group chooses a physician of your specialty.
   a. Types of referral include patient referral, physician referral, a combination of patient and physician referral, the phone book, hospital recommendation, and the sign outside the office.

b. It is important to understand the subtle differences in the way that patients choose their doctors. For example, in your practice you might find that women tend to choose their doctors based on a personal referral, while men tend to select on the basis of a telephone book listing. If this were the case, you might wish to change your telephone book advertising to increase its appeal to men, and stress a referral reinforcement program to thank those women who are referring patients to you.

5. Identify the method of transportation taken by the key groups to their doctor. For example, if you have many elderly patients who use public transportation and must walk a few blocks from the nearest bus stop, perhaps you could increase your patient flow by relocating your office closer to public transportation.

6. Determine the percentage of your patients who are covered by third-party payers. It is useful to know the overall percentage as well as the breakdown by different insurance companies; you should also evaluate the profitability by type of policy and the ease of collection from the insurer.

   a. Different insurance companies often pay different rates; in addition, some companies cover more types of procedures. You will want to determine whether one of the insurance companies used by your patients is better than others and begin to develop a marketing program to increase the proportion of patients with the better type of insurance.

   b. You might want to determine specifically how those patients covered by third parties are choosing your services and plan your marketing program accordingly.

7. Evaluate the demographic trends in your trade area and their potential impact on your practice.

   a. Is the population aging?
   b. Is there increasing unemployment?
   c. Is the birthrate increasing, stable, or declining?
   d. Are there growing numbers of families?
   e. Are spending habits changing?
   f. Has the occupational pattern been changing?

8. Research the current health delivery trends in your trade area.

   a. Health Maintenance Organization (HMO) activity
   b. Preferred Provider Organization (PPO) activity, including free-standing emergency clinics
   c. Hospital activity
   d. Group practices
   e. Business coalitions

    f. Third-party activity

    g. Patient coalitions and cooperatives

Assessing Your Competition

Competition in medicine, which may seem a distasteful concept, results from physician oversupply and from the involvement of organized groups in the formation of low-cost group practices. It is important to evaluate the effect of competition on your practice and to identify any provider who competes for your services directly in your area. You want to understand whether your area is oversupplied and why particular practices are growing while others are declining. You will also want to find out what complaints patients have about your competition (and compare those complaints with ones that have been noted in your practice).

The following questions should be considered in completing the part of your audit that analyzes competition.

1. Find out the ratio of patients to physicians in your trade area (that is, the total number of physicians in your defined trading area divided into the total population). Determine this ratio in your specialty.
2. Pinpoint all competition.
   a. Within your area.
   b. Outside of your area.
3. Identify which practices are growing and why.
4. Identify which practices are on the decline and why.
5. What are the key complaints of patients about doctors in your trade area?
6. Is there room for more doctors? How many?
7. What do your competitors charge?
8. What services do your competitors offer that you don't?
9. Have you assessed the size and business of your practices vis-à-vis your competition (market share)?

Assessing Your Practice Development

Each practice is unique and grows for unique reasons; you need to determine the development of your practice, the key milestones in its growth, and its overall strengths and weaknesses. Your objective in assessing your practice development will be to identify and continue to nurture the important aspects of your practice that contributed to its growth. Some topics that should be covered in your assessment are the following.

1. History
   a. When did your practice begin?
   b. Where was it first located?
   c. What were the key milestones in practice growth?
   d. How fast did the practice grow?
   e. How has your patient mix changed over the years?
   f. Why did your patients come to you?
   g. Why have your patients left you?
   h. How has your practice done financially? (your estimate against national average)
   i. What have been your major headaches? (staff? collections?)
2. Practice strengths and weaknesses
   a. Staff, including reception, nursing, and financial personnel.
   b. Facility—interior design, efficiency layout.
   c. Management ability—your own and that of your spouse and your advisors.
   d. Clinical and diagnostic skills.
   e. Specialized procedures.
   f. Specialized equipment.
   g. Personal reputation.
   h. Capitalization or financial strength.
   i. Your practice image in the community
3. Your staff
   a. Qualifications.
   b. Salaries.
   c. Attitude.
   d. Ability.
   e. Experience.
   f. Skills.
   g. Training.
   h. Personalities.
4. Your systems
   a. Appointments.
   b. Telephone handling.
   c. Collections.
   d. Patient management.
   e. Financial.
5. Dependency on outside factors
   a. Third-party influence.

      b. Industries.

      c. Competition (HMOs or other organizations).

      d. Medical society.

6. Organization

      a. Delegation.

      b. Patient orientation.

      c. Methods of addressing your weaknesses.

      d. Regularity, productivity, and effectiveness of staff meetings.

      e. Ease of implementing new systems, direction of policies.

7. Government and external controls

      a. Medical society.

      b. Peer pressure.

      c. Hospital.

      d. Federal, state, local government.

      e. Trends that affect your practice specifically.

Assessing The Way You Deliver Service

In the past, you practiced medicine without really analyzing what you did well and what perception your patients had of your service. In the competitive environment, as patients become more aware of their health care needs, a focus on patients' perceptions of your services will become crucial. It is also important to know which of the procedures and services you provide are profitable and which are not, and to determine what differentiates your services from those of other practitioners in your trade area.

Cost accounting will become critical in your decision-making process, as will the use of computers to assess your practice. With a comprehensive data base of your patients and an analysis of the use of services by diagnosis you will have the ability to target specific areas of your practice for growth.

In analyzing service delivery, remember the concept of augmented service—that is, most patients judge you by the way you appear to be and the way the practice is managed, since they do not have enough information to judge your skill as a physician. A well-managed practice will significantly improve your patients' perception of you.

The following are key questions to consider when developing an assessment of service delivery.

1. Do you know the top 30 procedures or services that account for 80 percent of your revenue?

2. Do you know your patients' perception of each service?

3. What differentiates your services and the way you deliver them from those of other physicians in your trade area that provide the same services?

4. Do you understand the relationship of each of your services to practice profitability?

5. Do you have an accurate cost accounting for each service and for your time, the staff's time, and supplies and equipment used?

6. What are the demographic characteristics of patients needing each service you perform?

7. What new services have you added as a result of patient demand, change in technology, and philosophy of your practice?

8. Have you assessed the trends in services delivered as your practice has developed?

9. What services have you been known for?

10. What do you do more of? Why?

11. What do you do less of? Why?

12. What key social, economic, and technological changes have impacted upon the services you deliver?

13. What are the most frequent positive comments about each service?

14. What are the most frequent negative comments about each service?

15. What new services should you be adding to attract, keep, or satisfy patients?

16. How much of your time is spent specifically performing procedures?

17. Is one procedure more profitable or less profitable than the next?

18. Have you highlighted your practice attributes to your patients to give you an edge over the competition?

Assessing Your Fees and Pricing Strategies

The area of fee-setting will be one that will undergo a significant amount of change in the competitive era. Health-maintenance organizations spearheaded the concept of a fixed monthly payment for all medical services; this trend toward fixed reimbursement services will continue to grow. Hospitals are already being reimbursed through diagnostically related groups—that is, a hospital will receive a fixed fee for a specific diagnosis. This trend will affect physician reimbursement in the future. The idea of fixed fees is taking hold because patients like the idea of knowing specifically what the cost for health care will be so that it can be budgeted on a monthly basis.

Physicians have rarely surveyed their competition regarding their fees, and they have applied a relatively arbitrary formula to fee setting. In the future, as patients become more price sensitive, the process of setting fees will be one that we will have to spend more time on than we did in the past.

As third-party payers begin to base their fees on the diagnosis combined with the severity of illness, we will see a proliferation of different fee strategies. In the past, the private-practice fee-for-service physician charged what he felt was fair and reasonable for the patient. In the future there will be more intervention from third parties regarding this issue.

It is important for physicians to assess and understand the different methods for setting and charging fees as different methods of payment established by insurance companies and government begin to affect the way that services are delivered. Physicians may find themselves practicing particular brands or styles of medicine in specific geographic areas; significant practice losses may occur if they do not understand the subtleties of reimbursement that affect their practice. They should review their fee structures at least on a quarterly basis on the basis of the profitability of the services. Changing overhead costs should be monitored and then reflected in fee changes.

Some questions to consider when assessing your fees within the marketing audit are the following:

1. Policies upon which to base your fee level
   a. Relative value—Blue Shield schedule
   b. Personal relative value scales (weighting the different services you prefer)
   c. Cost plus
   d. Base price plus extras
   e. Market pricing
   f. Value pricing
   g. Loss leaders (for example, the $25 physical)
2. Frequency of change.
   a. Annually, biannually, or quarterly.
   b. Overhead monitoring reflected in fee changes.
3. Levels of increase for the past five years
4. Reactions to Fee Changes by
   a. Your patients.
   b. Your competitors.

c. Third-party payers.
d. Government.

Assessing Your Patient Communication and Promotion

The communication and promotional aspects of the practice have been left to last, since it is usually the last thing you should consider in your medical practice audit. Communication and promotion are, however, an integral part of the patient education process. Together they are the dominant influence on how your patients perceive your practice.

In a competitive environment your communication and practice promotion will be highly scrutinized by your patients. It is critical to develop an appropriate communications plan; in time you will have to become more aggressive in your promotion to stay viable.

An integral part of your promotional program is your advertising and referral reinforcement programs, which are, in turn, closely tied in with developing a practice image and style congruent with the expectations of your patients. Here are a number of key items to consider when developing this part of your medical practice market audit.

1. How effective is patient education?
   a. Credit policy.
   b. Patient recalls and reminders.
   c. Follow through on course of treatment.
   d. New patient inquiries.
   e. First visit.
2. What new methods have been introduced and tried within the past five years?
   a. Successes.
   b. Failures?
3. What are the current advertising and public relations strategy?
   a. Yellow pages.
   b. Business cards.
   c. Practice brochures.
   d. Patient handout materials.
   e. Public speaking.
   f. Radio and television talk shows.
4. How aggressive is the competition in treatment of paid forms, advertising, and patient solicitations?
5. What patient referral reinforcement programs do you have in effect?
   a. Thank you letters.

      b. Personal calls.

      c. Notation in charts.

      d. Christmas cards, and so on.

  6. What statistics are in place to monitor promotional effectiveness?

  7. Have you assessed your own image, style, and persuasiveness? Can it be improved? How? What are you doing about it?

Assessing Your Location and Availability

From a marketing perspective, your location and availability are essential aspects of the concept of access to services. The easier it is for a patient to see you because of a convenient location or availability of appointments, the better it will be for your practice. Patient demands will become more critical in the future as their alternative choices for health care grow.

The following are some of key considerations when you study location. The whole issue of location is addressed in more depth in a later chapter; however, we will touch on it here since it is a critical part of the market audit.

  1. What are the current trends in your trading area?

      a. Free-standing centers.

      b. Mobile services.

      c. Evening and Saturday hours.

      d. Shopping mall locations.

      e. Twenty-four hour service facilities.

  2. What trends exist in your specialty for part-time or satellite clinics in the region?

  3. How great is the demand for evening and weekend hours?

Assessing Your Opportunities

In developing a marketing plan, after the market audit it is important to consider the availability of opportunities for practice growth and success. To do this effectively you will have to weigh the risks versus the rewards of each opportunity. For example, a full-page advertisement in the newspaper may bring in a number of patients to your practice and make you very successful. The risk, however, is that you may lose the respect of your colleagues. In looking at each opportunity, you should consider both the risks and the rewards; making a good decision involves balancing both factors.

The issues of expansion and affiliation with other physicians to preserve your practices will become more critical. Physicians are already affiliating with other physicians to pool promotional and management resources and to offer longer hours, so that they can remain competitive.

As hospitals become more involved in the success of medical practices, hospital affiliation with medical staffs and joint ventures between them become more important. Hospitals are typically well financed and their success largely depends on the success of their medical staff, and affiliation between physicians and hospitals will become closer. Hospitals are already offering management advice and capital to allow their medical staff to compete more effectively in the marketplace. This trend will continue, and we have already seen hospitals throughout the nation closing their medical staff and consolidating their operations in cooperation with their medical staff.

When developing this aspect of the plan, you must weigh risks against rewards and evaluate the usefulness of expansion or affiliation with other physicians, hospitals, or national coalitions. To develop a successful practice, you will need to take a hard look at where you have been, where you are now, and where you are going. By completing the medical practice audit and committing it to paper, reviewing it periodically, and updating it annually, you will be better able to survive the competitive challenges of the future.

●

Chapter 4

Pricing Strategies

The pricing of your services previously required little attention. At the end of the year the typical physician met with his or her accountant to review the overall costs of delivering services to patients; if those costs had increased the physician would raise the fees accordingly to cover expenses and build in a margin of profit. In this traditional cost-centered approach to the pricing of medical services, little time was spent in reviewing pricing policies or in evaluating the management of this aspect of medical practice. In a competitive era, however, pricing strategy becomes more crucial; if poorly addressed, it can cause you to lose a number of patients to your competition.

Patients attitudes are being sensitized now more than ever to the cost of health care. This is being accomplished in large urban areas through regular radio and television advertising by health maintenance organizations (HMOs) stressing the desirability of their pricing strategy; in addition, the national media attention received from government discussions on containing national health care costs sensitizes the patients' awareness to fees. Now more than ever, patients are interested in how the costs of services are being computed.

The once-held notion that price is not a determining factor in how patients choose their doctors is being challenged with the new patient attitude. If you believe that your fees are not a determining factor in a patient's choice of a doctor, you might have a rude awakening. In highly competitive areas such as Portland, Oregon, doctors daily receive calls from patients who are price shopping for medical care and comparing prices between practices. This is a trend that is sure to continue as the physician oversupply grows throughout the country. As the health care market place becomes more competitive, you will begin to see a number of creative pricing strategies emerging to capitalize on this marketing opportunity.

A recent phenomenon is the fixed-price strategy being promoted by a number of groups and physicians throughout the country with a great deal of success. The HMOs, for example, offer a fixed price for medical services; that is, for a fixed monthly premium, patients have all their health care needs covered if they restrict themselves to a particular group of doctors and hospitals. Patients like HMOs for many reasons. The fixed cost for care is a desirable idea, patients have no insurance forms to fill out, they can begin to budget health as a regular monthly expense, and they have no additional charges to cope with.

A fixed-price strategy involving doctors in private practice has developed in California to counter the HMO trend. One pediatrician near San Francisco adopted a fixed-price system in his private practice. The parents paid a set fee of about $300 for all the well-baby check-ups in the first year. They paid $60 down and $20 per month, and could bring the child in as many times as necessary during the first year as well as call in for advice. There has been a very favorable response from patients to this method, which is working very well.

A further private practice strategy to counter the HMOs is the approach of the individual practice association (IPA), in which private practitioners contract with a marketing group to provide services as independent practitioners to patients requiring this type of service. Some medical practices may have privately paying patients who represent half of his practice; the other half of the practice would be IPA patients from whom the doctor would get a fixed monthly fee for taking care of their needs. IPAs have not been as successful in their marketing efforts since they are usually not as aggressive in their promotion as HMOs.

With the implementation of diagnostic related groups (DRGs) as a pricing mechanism in hospitals, price competition based on fixed reimbursements is being forced onto hospitals by government and business. DRGs are a method of reimbursement to hospitals based on diagnosis. Briefly, a hospital would be paid a fixed price for an appendicectomy, for example. Since there is no incentive to increase the length of stay in the hospital, the emphasis would be on efficiency and effectiveness. I predict that if pricing based on diagnosis works in hospitals then it will be brought into the private medical sector. This type of pricing is being tested for potential implementation as a reimbursement method for private practice in the future.

If private practitioners want the fee-for-service approach to succeed as a pricing strategy, more effort should be given to thinking through the positive approaches to this way of pricing.

Some physicians are taking creative approaches to pricing, including the base price plus extras approach. One application of this approach involves alternatives to the annual physical—for example, the base price for an annual physical could be $65, which would include the basic tests and work-up. For $150 the patient receives the basic physical plus more tests and more time spent with the doctor, and for $300 he or she gets even more tests and more time spent with the doctor and staff. Different people perceive themselves as needing different levels of health care; as a result, those that have the finances and the interest in a $300 physical should be able to purchase it from you.

As you become sensitized to the fact that patients have different levels of health expectation, you should extend the same thinking to analyzing how your patients perceive the rest of your fees.

Patients seem most aware of the cost of your average office call or consultation; you should be very sensitive to price fluctuations and changes in this fee. Because your service may be measured based on the cost of this fee, you should pay close attention to prevailing local fees in this area.

Discount medicine has had negative connotations that have steered many practitioners away from this approach. There are many reasons why you might want to offer discounts in your practice, and they may be desirable when competing with other low-cost pricing strategies. One good use of discount pricing is the concept of giving a discount for cash at the time of service. It costs you about $2 to send a bill to a patient; therefore if the patient pays cash at the time of service, this saves you that amount. A number of physicians offer this as a discount or half of this discount to a patient, because this improves collections and can increase your net income.

Another pricing strategy that will emerge involves establishing a differential for additional patient amenities. The service industry for a long period of time has recognized the difference in consumers' requirements for service. On an airplane, for example, you can fly coach or first class—both methods get you to the same destination and the core service provided is the same. The augmented services, or customer amenities, in first class are significantly better, however; these amenities include wider seats, more contact with hostesses, and improved meals. Similarly, a medical office offers one level of core service, but more patient amenities could be offered to those who are prepared to pay for them. Patients requesting first-class service in a medical practice would be booked during choice appointment times. Extra staff could be in the office during these times, physicians might spend more personal time with these particular patients, and extra patient handouts and educational materials might be given since they are paying extra. A patient seeing the doctor with a complaint could request either first-class service or normal service. The patient would receive the same quality of core service, with the same diagnosis and the same treatment methods, but the augmented services and the special touches would be in the first-class service.

Many physicians wonder whether they should set high prices for their services because people may perceive that higher prices are associated with better service. This idea holds true if you are prepared to offer the additional patient amenities required for a higher level of service as you would provide in first class. By placing your fees at a high level, you will attract those patients looking for additional patient amenities and service. If these amenities and services are not provided, pricing strategy will not succeed in the long run. Your objective should be to price your services appropriately based on the level of service you want to provide.

As we move into the new pricing era, it is important to ensure that your prices are well thought out and relate to an audit of practices in the area; you must pay particular attention to setting your fees appropriately if you expect your practice enhancement program to succeed in this consumer environment.

●

Chapter 5

Assessing Your Location: A Key Ingredient in Practice Success

In a competitive era your success will be influenced by three important variables: location, location, and location. In the past, you could locate your practice virtually in a tree house and patients would beat a path to your door. Times have changed, however; physicians now have to compete—and the right location can make the difference between success and failure. The competitive pressure has led to storefront medical offices in shopping malls, free-standing facilities in high-traffic locations, mobile medical offices, and other creative location strategies.

This chapter addresses the question of practice location. Whether you are an established physician considering relocating your practice or setting up a satellite, or a new doctor about to select an office location for the first time, the principles in location analysis are the same.

We will start by looking at some general principles for assessing a region. We will then move to specific methods to evaluate the demographic characteristics of a location and finally to methods on how to pinpoint a specific area to locate a practice.

The choice of choosing a general geographic location in which to practice has always been a trade off between patient demand and personal and family considerations. Doctors have traditionally been advised to choose a region where they would be happiest practicing, and then consider the patient demand situation in the area; times have changed, however. To succeed in the future, you will have to pay closer attention to patient demographic trends and physician manpower needs. You might even have to consider relocating your practice or setting up a satellite in a more desirable suburb or more visible location to continue to be viable.

Many surveys have indicated that patients feel their doctors' offices are not located conveniently enough for their needs. Although patients will travel long distances to see their doctors—out of loyalty and habit—this will begin to change as convenience and travel costs begin to outweigh the importance of the traditional physician-patient personal relationship.

A number of factors need to be considered before you make your final decision on a reason to locate. You must balance patient demand for personal satisfaction. Factors to consider include:

1. Proximity to medical education and teaching centers
2. Nearness to family and friends
3. Cultural opportunities of interest to you and your spouse
4. Educational system for your children
5. Size of the community
6. Distance to hospitals
7. Quality of recreational opportunities available
8. Climate

With these key considerations in mind, I would recommend that you go where you are needed.

Table 5-1 shows a suggested ratio of patients to practitioner by specialty area. These numbers were extrapolated from my experience working with a number of physicians and should be used only as a general guideline. Issues of utilization, orientation to prevention, and referral patterns significantly affect the need for various patient services. For example, in rural and farming communities patients go to their doctors less often than urban dwellers, who are believers in preventive medicine. However, this will give you a good base to start. The American Medical Association's state and county medical societies can give you specific data on manpower planning for your analysis.

As a sample application of the information in Table 5-1, assume that you are an internist who would like to locate in Desirable City, California. Your first move would be to obtain the most recent yellow pages of that city's telephone book or to ask the local Medical Society for the number

Figure 5-1

PRACTICE LOCATION WORKSHEET	Site 1	Site 2	Site 3
Name, address, phone number			
A. Office Type —Medical arts building, office complex, strip mall, enclosed mall, single office, house			
B. Area —Urban core, central business district, secondary business district, string street development, neighborhood —Suburban —Undesirable neighbors (yes/no)			
C. Location —Convenience to patients —Convenience to hospitals —Staff privileges at new hospitals —Public transportation —Access to highways —Rush hour traffice congestion			
D. Character of building —Is building easy to find? —Does it have a professional appearance? —Does landlord have good reputation? —Is building well managed?			

E. Office Facilities: Specifics
—Parking
  on premises
  reasonable rates
  adjacent
  on street
  metered			

—Examing rooms (No.)			
—Bathrooms on premises off premises but convenient			
—Waiting room (sq. ft.)			
—Business office space (sq. ft.)			
—Storage space (sq. ft.)			
—Clinic area (sq. ft.)			
—Soundproof perimeter walls			
F. Utilities and services			
—Heating			
—Air-conditioning controlled from within outside control			
—Electric wiring capacity			
—Electric outlets (No. per room)			
—Janitorial service (No. hrs. avail.)			
—Monthly window washing			
—Light bulb replacement			
—Garbage removal			
—Elevator (adequate service)			
—Security			
—Partitioning included			
—Decoration allowance			
G. Financing			
—Terms ($ per sq. ft. per yr.)			
—Monthly rental			
—Annual increment			
—Period of lease			
—Option to renew			
—Option to sublet			
—Escape clause			
—Addit. comments			

Table 5-1. Estimated Physician: Population Ratios for Successful Practice.

Allergy	1 :	22,000–26,000
Anesthesiology	1 :	16,000–21,000
Family practice	1 :	1,700– 3,000
General surgery	1 :	8,000–12,000
Internal medicine	1 :	4,000– 6,000
Neurology	1 :	40,000–80,000
Neurosurgery	1 :	60,000–80,000
Obstetrics and gynecology	1 :	10,000–13,000
Ophthalmology	1 :	20,000–25,000
Orthopedics	1 :	30,000–35,000
Otolaryngology	1 :	35,000–45,000
Pathology	1 :	19,000–25,000
Pediatrics	1 :	8,000–12,000
Plastic surgery	1 :	40,000–60,000
Psychiatry	1 :	10,000–12,000
Radiology	1 :	14,000–17,000
Urology	1 :	30,000–40,000

of internists practicing in that area. If the general population of Desirable City is 500,000, using Table 5-1, we know that the Desirable City area could support 100 internists (assuming the ratio of 1 : 5,000).

You must also examine the statistics of related specialties. For example, if there are a number of family practitioners in an area, this will decrease the demand for internists' services; however, an area low in related specialties will have a greater population base to support you. If there are 100 or fewer internists practicing in Desirable City, then it is a relatively good area for an internist to locate. More often than not, however, you will find an urban area is well supplied with physicians in most specialities. Does this mean, then, that if the Desirable City area has more than 100 internists it cannot support another? The answer is no—provided that you do your demographic analysis properly. What it does tell you is that it will not be easy for an internist to succeed in Desirable City unless he or she intelligently selects the right location, as discussed in the following sections.

Pinpoint a Target Area

Go to the city hall planning office and purchase a large map of the area. Take some pins with colored heads and, by referring again to the yellow pages of the telephone book, pin the map where internists are located. This can be an enjoyable job for your children (if they are past the age of swallowing pins); it is a tedious, time-consuming task making sure the map has been properly pinned, but it is quite worthwhile. After the pinning process has been completed, you'll usually find that the internists are clustered in areas. A number of areas will have no pins, however, indicating potential opportunities. If your practice relies on referrals, use pins of a different color to indicate referral sources. Then talk with the potential referring physician to see whether he would refer patients to you if you were to locate your practice in that area.

Determine the Need for Your Services

In order to make a wise decision about an area that looks promising, you will need to do your homework. Specifically, your goal will be to uncover patient needs for medical services to which you can respond appropriately. For example, through some basic research, a new family physician in Ohio identified a need for evening and weekend hours, and that need was not being satisfied by local doctors. As a result, when he opened his practice he scheduled his daytime appointments on Mondays and Fridays only, since these were the busiest days, and the rest of his hours on evenings and Saturdays. His practice boomed right from the beginning, even though the town seemed to have too many family practitioners.

If you determine that the average age of the patient population is 45 and mainly male, for example, you would locate, furnish, staff, and deliver your services in a different way than if the average age of your patients was 28, and mostly female. Men prefer chairs with arms, *Sports Illustrated, Mechanics Illustrated,* and *Esquire* magazines in a masculine setting. Women, on the other hand, would prefer *Ms magazine, House & Garden,* and chairs without arms, in a traditionally more subtle feminine decor.

Other techniques used by professional location consultants include measuring automobile traffic flow and pedestrian traffic flow. Talk with your local city planning officials for automobile traffic counts, which will tell you how busy various streets are and will also give you a good reading on how many patients will be passing your location. Foot traffic or pedestrian counts are more difficult to obtain, but you can do them yourself by counting the number of pedestrians who pass a particular location in a five-minute period during each business day. These counts can be analyzed in terms of the number and type of people walking by your (potential) office. Traffic counts provide a strong indication of the possible volume of patients and how quickly your practice will grow.

It is also important to determine whether the traffic is on "your" side of the street or the other side. It is well documented that people generally walk on the sunny side. Of two competing businesses providing the same services, one could boom and the other go bankrupt, mainly because it was located on the "wrong" side of the street.

Assess the Growth Potential

After you have determined the need for your services, it is important to ensure that you are locating in a stable economic environment. When determining the economic characteristics of a region, watch for the following danger signs:

1. High school and college graduates generally must leave the region to find suitable employment.
2. Unemployment rates are high.
3. Retail sales and industrial production are declining.
4. Company bankruptcy rates are high.
5. Businessmen and academics have an apathetic attitude toward the region.

In contrast, these signs indicate more generally favorable conditions:

1. Chain or department stores are opening.
2. Branch plants are locating in the area.
3. Good transportation exists to all parts of the area.
4. There is a progressive industrial commission.
5. Business and residential premises are well maintained.
6. Construction activity is increasing.

Do Your Demographic Analysis

There are a number of excellent sources of demographic information available to you. Local municipalities often have an industrial commission that can provide more current community data, collected to attract industry into the area. You can obtain this information by writing to the industrial commissioner in the particular area.

Most larger urban areas have a Chamber of Commerce, which can give you helpful facts and statistics about the communty. Health planning councils also collect information on patient demographic characteristics, which can be obtained from the local council.

Whether you are setting up your practice for the first time, planning to establish a satellite, or thinking about relocating, doing this demographic homework is critical. If you are an established practitioner, you might feel that you know enough about the area to make this decision. However, it is my suggestion that you take a systematic approach based on the numbers presented. You might be surprised to find that the demographic characteristics of your patients differs widely from the norm in the area. Your aim will be to make a decision based on objective criteria, and that means you will have to do your homework.

Other methods of procuring information include the following:

1. Take license numbers from parked cars in your area and determine the owners' addresses from the Transportation department.

2. If you are locating in a suburb or a large town, find out the total circulation of the local newspaper and that will give you a good idea what the "drawing" area is.

3. Ask local businessmen and bankers from what territory they draw their customers and depositors.

Determine Specific Needs

By this time, you should have volumes of information about your community. Look at the map you pinned and identify the underserved areas. Do some specific research to determine patient needs. This might include a simple telephone survey of random patients, asking for specific feedback and opinions on medical services presently being offered. Some questions might be: What do you like or dislike about medical services in your area? Are the hours convenient? What changes would you like to see in physician services?

It may be a good learning experience to do the survey yourself, even if it means conducting it anonymously by telephone. When you study the results of the survey, pay very close attention to patient complaints about their present medical services. Also, make note of what physicians with large and successful practices are doing. Perhaps they are filling a special need that you too could fill. Look for practices with innovative ideas and try to apply these ideas to your practice.

The Final Details Needed to Assess a Location

Having chosen your general locality, you must determine your specific practice location. Figure 5-1 is a checklist of considerations to keep in mind when weighing the alternatives. Key points to consider are:

1. Is it convenient and acceptable to patients?
2. Is it on a bus line?
3. Is there ample parking without worrying about parking meters?
4. Is the office near the hospital or other medical facilities?
5. Is it possible to get an on-call group together?
6. Is it fairly close to your home?

Generally speaking, if you are a specialist and you spend a lot of time at the hospital, you will locate your practice as close to the hospital as possible. If you are a primary care physician, you will need to locate near your patient base.

Chapter 6

Referral Management: A Critical Variable in Practice Growth and Success

In the past, a physician rarely worried about patients leaving his or her practice. Since the supply of physicians did not meet the demand, there was always a steady stream of new patients that could replace those leaving. Therefore, there was very little need to invest time and effort in managing referrals for practice growth.

As competition increases, it is more important to expand your current patient referral base. Since most practices grow largely as a result of word-of-mouth advertising, a referral managing program is crucial in sustaining practice growth in this competitive era. Can you name the top ten referral sources for your practice? What have you done recently to acknowledge their contribution to the growth and success of your practice? The answers to these questions can only be made after a careful study of your referral statistics. You need to establish who your referral sources are and monitor your practice growth (the actual monitoring process is detailed in depth in the next chapter).

A referral management report, as shown in Figure 6-1, allows you to

52

Figure 6-1

Referral Sources Analysis

	Jan.	Feb.	Mar.	Apr.	May	June	July	Aug.	Sept.	Oct.	Nov.	Dec.
M.D.'s												
Name												
Name												
Name												
Hospital A												
Hospital B												
Yellow Pages												
Walk-ins												
Lecture												
Radio												
TV												
Newspaper												
School Nurses												
Name												
Name												
Clergy												
Industrial Nurses												
Name												
Service Clubs												
Patients												
Name												
Name												
Name												
Name												
Name												
Name												
Name												
Name												
Referrals												
Secondary Referrals												
Personal Friends												
Name												
Name												
Total Referrals												

make a detailed list of each of your referral sources. If you are in a specialty practice you need to include both physicians who refer patients to you and your own patients who refer their friends or relatives. Any lectures, radio, or television work should be noted as referral sources so that you can determine how these activities contribute to your marketing program.

Thanking Your Referral Sources

The acknowledgment of referral sources is extremely important in building referrals. When you see a new patient who was referred by a colleague or by another patient, you should try to thank your sources in as many ways as you can.

All patient referrals should be noted specifically in a chart, and you should keep an ongoing list of patients who have referred others. A letter or thank you card should be generated for each new patient referred. I recommend sending a separate letter to a physician source thanking him or her specifically for the referral, rather than integrating it with the consultation letter.

When there have been several referrals from one source, you should think of more creative ways of thanking that individual. If the source is one of your patients, you can make a note in that patient's chart that he or she is referring to the practice; you should also thank him or her at the next check-up or other visit. Colleagues who have referred several patients should be thanked personally when you encounter them.

By keeping a list of the names and addresses of referral sources, you will be able to remember them during the holidays, and you may wish to send greetings for birthdays and other special occasions. You might also consider inviting all your referral sources to a special Christmas party or other holiday celebration. This reinforces your confidence in them and is a way of maintaining regular contact.

Patients That Leave You

Patients leave your practice for different reasons—many of them are moving away but some are dissatisfied with the service. Either you or your nurse should talk to each patient leaving your practice to determine the reasons for the change. Specific complaints should be noted, and you should try to act on any of them that seem to reflect legitimate problems with the service you are rendering. Your objective will be to minimize the problems within your practice and maximize the positive aspects.

A crucial aspect of your referral management program demands that you list the referral sources for patients who leave your practice. Are these patients being referred from a specific physician? This could involve an incompatibility problem with a particular physician. Perhaps patients are used to a specific level of service with one doctor and have certain expectations from you that you are not fulfilling. You must also remember that as patients leave they go back to their referring source and can begin to change that person's opinion of you. Therefore it is critical that you analyze the records of these patients to determine if there are any patterns that related back to the referring source.

Telephone Contact

By knowing all patients who currently perceive you as their doctor and determining why patients enter your practice and why they leave, you will have set in motion a process that will pay dividends in practice growth. Counting your patients is not enough, however—you and your staff must express enthusiasm, warmth, and gratitude to your patients. One way of doing this is to let your patients know you are thinking about them by making a call once in a while from your practice to see how they are. You could hire a student once or twice a year to call patients and update records (this would also give you good information for your patient retention program).

─────────────────────────●

Chapter 7

Patient Accounting: A Method for Managing Practice Growth

Patient accounting means exactly that—accounting for every patient who comes into or leaves your practice. This means that you need to pay close attention to changes in patient volume, new patients, and service mix. You do this by gathering daily, weekly, and monthly statistics and monitoring and assessing changes as they occur. The term *service mix* refers to the types of services you might be performing; for example, if you are an ophthalmologist, you will be doing more cataract surgery if your average patient age is 50 rather than 30 years.

The Value of Patient Accounting

Patient accounting has many benefits. First, it lets you know precisely whether your practice is growing, remaining stable, or declining. It also puts you in better control of your practice's patient flow, since you know how many patients and what types of patients you are seeing, thus allowing you to develop your ideal practice situation. Patient accounting can, in addition, let you know the general mix of different types of procedures you are doing, giving you historical data to project into the future. Moreover, it keeps track of new patients—the lifeblood of your practice—and who referred them to you. It also keeps an account of patients who leave the practice and why.

Recent surveys I have made of thousands of patients indicate that by far the largest determinant of practice growth is patient referral. Whether you are in a primary care practice or a specialty, your ultimate success in the competitive marketplace will be determined through patient referrals. In a surgical practice, the majority of your referrals during your first five years will come from other physicians. As you become more established, referrals from patients begin to outnumber those from physicians. In a primary care practice, satisfied patients will refer their friends. This is by far the best method of building any successful service establishment, and a medical practice is in the business of servicing patients.

Critical to the viability and success of a practice in this competitive era is a mechanism to monitor practice growth and patient referrals. Such monitoring is not possible without specific procedures. An example of what can happen without such procedures can be seen in the practice of a general surgeon who was proud of having 17,253 patient records on file. Although a lot of hard work and long hours had gone into building the patient roster, the doctor did not know how many patients had moved away or died, and most important, how and why the patients had sought out his practice initially.

Most medical practices grow in many different ways. Few physicians know precisely why patients have come to their practice, why they leave, and who specifically referred them to there—or, even more important, why they were chosen by the referral source.

What Is Patient Accounting?

Patient accounting is a system of monitoring your patients, who are your most valuable assets. You should treat them as such and account for each one of them, just as you monitor your financial assets, liabilities, expenses, and revenues through financial accounting systems. You need to understand how your patients view the positive attributes (assets) of your practice, as well as the negative characteristics (liabilities); moreover, you need to monitor how these attributes affect patient flow.

Figure **7-1**

Patient Referral Report

Patients Seen	Sun	Mon	Tue	Wed	Thur	Fri	Sat	TOTAL
1. Office visits								
2. Surgical procedures								
3. Consultations								
4. Emergency room								
5. Miscellaneous								
TOTAL PATIENTS SEEN								
Patient Mix								
New patients								
Patients leaving								
Return patients								
TOTAL PATIENT CHARTS								
Referral Sources								
1. M.D.s								
2. Our Patients								
3. Hosp. A (who)								
4. Hosp. B (who)								
5. Other hospitals (which, who)								
6. Walk-ins								
7. Lecture								
8. Radio, TV								
9. Newspaper								
10. School nurses								
11. Industrial nurses								
12. Service clubs								
13. Other								

Implementing Patient Accounting in Your Practice

Figure 7-1 is an example of a typical patient accounting report—the heart of the patient accounting system (of course, you will customize the form to adapt to your own circumstances). Figure 7-2 shows a form used to list patients who leave a practice.

Each day, from your day sheets and appointment book, you should note how many patients you saw in the office, how many surgical or other procedures were done, and other miscellaneous related data. It is critical that you compare the number of new patients with the number of patients leaving, and note the total under your care at that particular time. To determine how many active patients you have, add up all the

Figure 7-2

**Patients Leaving Practice
Report**

For Period of _____

Patient Name	Doctor	Service Rendered	Patient Reaction	Reason for Leaving

charts of those who have been in to see you within the last three years. These are your active charts.

Set up a specific sheet on each referral source, and every time that source refers a patient to you, note it on the sheet. These should be compared on a regular basis to see whether referrals are increasing, remaining stable, or declining. The total number of patients from your referral sources should be noted under the heading Referral Sources in Figure 7-1. You can obtain a great deal of information regarding your referral sources by having your medical assistant ask new patients how they heard about you.

If you have a patient introduction form, or a form that patients sign in with (giving their name, address, telephone number, and so forth), you can ask the questions on that form: "Who referred you to this practice?" and "Do you know anyone else who comes to this practice?" Questions can be worded in such a way that patients provide their own demographic information.

Some specialty practices pay students to call the patients directly. The caller states that the office is updating charts to make sure all information is correct. Patients who no longer go to your practice or who no longer consider you their doctor will say so at this time.

The patient accounting system is a basis for gathering information on your practice's growth. As you gather statistics over a period of time, you will begin to develop a profile of your practice. For example, if surgical procedures normally account for 33 percent of your patient volume, you can consider it a warning sign if surgery has dropped to 10 percent of your overall volume. The next step would be to investigate why your surgical practice is declining.

Critical to practice growth is the influx of new patients. You will always want to have more patients coming into your practice than leaving. Sometimes a busy physician might think it sensible to close his or her practice to new patients. The volume of the practice will, however, decline significantly after a few years. There may be a demand for the services of the physician, but many of the original patients will have moved away and no new patients are filling the openings. I always recommend keeping a waiting list for your practice; as patients leave, one can fill in with new patients from this list.

Utilizing the Referral Sources Statistics

Monitoring your referral sources is especially critical in specialty practices. Since the majority of the referrals come from other doctors, monitoring increases and decreases in referrals becomes critical. One radiologist who was monitoring referrals found that one of his top ten referral sources had stopped sending patients to him. Later during a discussion in the doctors' lounge, he found out that his receptionist had been rude to the referring doctor when he called in. The receptionist was fired immediately, and the highly regarded referral source resumed sending patients to the radiologist's practice.

Another use of the referral source statistics is to acknowledge your referrals. Experts in practice building say that the acknowledgment of your referrals sources is the key ingredient to the growth of a practice. Every time a new patient is referred to your practice, whether through a physician, patient, or other member of the community, you should send a thank you letter specifically related to the referral. Some physicians note all referral sources in their patient records and thank patients personally each time they direct a friend to the practice.

By regularly tabulating, interpreting, and acting on the information retrieved from referral statistics, you will be taking a positive step toward managing the successful growth of your practice.

●

Chapter 8

Questionnaires and Other Types of Feedback from Patients

Keeping your patients satisfied means knowing what they're satisfied about, what they like about your practice, and what they dislike about it. An effective, yet inexpensive way to elicit patient feedback is through the implementation of a patient survey mechanism. Figure 8-1 shows a sample patient survey that you might find of interest. By surveying your patients about the various aspects of your practice, you'll find that you will get good response to successful aspects of your practice and indications of areas that need improvement. Any time response to surveys deviates from your standard, you will know that you should start asking questions. A more thorough evaluation with an in-depth questionnaire, which should be done at least once a year, can obtain demographic information and answers to more specific questions regarding various aspects of the practice.

Regular feedback from your patients regarding various practice management aspects of your clinic will motivate your staff to action and allow you to anticipate any potential problems. If your receptionist's courtesy and responsiveness are waning, your patients will be the first

Figure **8-1**

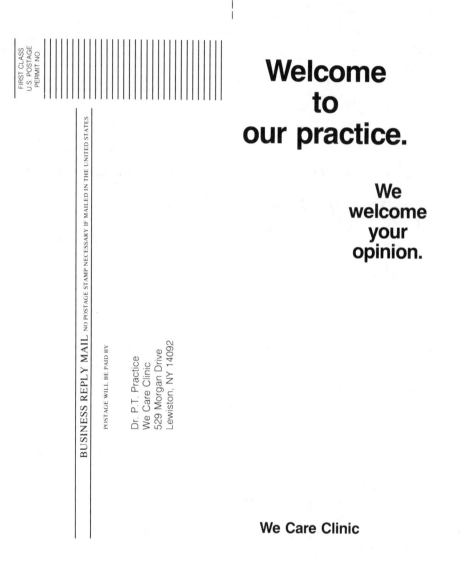

FIRST CLASS
U.S. POSTAGE
PERMIT NO.

BUSINESS REPLY MAIL NO POSTAGE STAMP NECESSARY IF MAILED IN THE UNITED STATES

POSTAGE WILL BE PAID BY

Dr. P.T. Practice
We Care Clinic
529 Morgan Drive
Lewiston, NY 14092

Welcome
to
our practice.

We
welcome
your
opinion.

We Care Clinic

We Care Clinic

To our valued patient:

Welcome to our practice. We are pleased to have you as a patient and will do our best to serve you well.

We strive to deliver the level of service that you expect from your doctor. To do this, we ask for your help. We value your comments and want to hear about the things we do right, and the things we need to improve.

Thank you for taking the time to complete this card.

Sincerely,

Dr. P.T. Practice

To help us make your future visits to our office comfortable and pleasant . . . please indicate how you feel about the following:

	Poor	Fair	Good	Very Good	Excellent
Telephone handling					
Courtesy & responsiveness of receptionist.	☐	☐	☐	☐	☐
Ease of appointment handling	☐	☐	☐	☐	☐
Being placed on hold	☐	☐	☐	☐	☐
Your reception on arrival (reception staff)					
Your greeting on arrival	☐	☐	☐	☐	☐
Fast & efficient check-in	☐	☐	☐	☐	☐
Comfort & cleanliness of reception area	☐	☐	☐	☐	☐
Was your welcome . . .	☐	☐	☐	☐	☐
The clinical assistants (nursing staff)					
Courteous & friendly	☐	☐	☐	☐	☐
Thoroughness	☐	☐	☐	☐	☐
Efficiency	☐	☐	☐	☐	☐
Responsive to your needs	☐	☐	☐	☐	☐
Your appointment					
At a convenient time	☐	☐	☐	☐	☐
Length of wait in office to see Doctor	☐	☐	☐	☐	☐
Pleasantness of wait	☐	☐	☐	☐	☐

Your time with doctor

Length of time spent	☐	☐	☐	☐	☐
Did the doctor listen to you & understand your problem	☐	☐	☐	☐	☐
Thoroughness of the exam	☐	☐	☐	☐	☐
Your questions answered	☐	☐	☐	☐	☐

Your doctor

Knowledge & ability to keep up with new methods & ideas	☐	☐	☐	☐	☐
Friendly & courteous	☐	☐	☐	☐	☐
Compassionate & caring	☐	☐	☐	☐	☐
Attentive to your needs	☐	☐	☐	☐	☐

Miscellaneous

Convenience of our location	☐	☐	☐	☐	☐
Overall personal attention received	☐	☐	☐	☐	☐

Any suggestions to improve our service to you would be appreciated.

to know about it. In many practices it might take six months for you to find out that the service has declined in this area.

Generally speaking, 80 percent of the responses to the survey should fall into the categories very good or excellent. If 20 percent or more of the responses are poor to fair, it indicates that your service is below standard.

The feedback mechanisms also allow your patients to express their feelings if they have a negative experience in the practice. Rather than take the unfortunate step of leaving your practice, they can take an active step by letting you know their thoughts through the feedback card. This allows you the opportunity to respond to the patient or remedy the problem. You should encourage patients to put their names and addresses on their communications so you can reach them about complaints. A stamped, self-addressed envelope marked "confidential" will encourage the patient feedback.

When a problem has been reported, one of your medical assistants should fill out a form with the patient's name and the specific problem (a sample of such a form is seen in Figure 8-2); this form is used to ensure that the problem is acted upon. Any action that is taken and the final resolution of the problem are noted on the form at the applicable time. This use of problem follow-through forms, combined with the other forms of feedback, will allow your practice to monitor patients' satisfaction.

Figure **8-2**

Patient Problem Follow-Through Form

Patient Name and Address: _____

_____

The Reported Problem

_____

_____

_____

_____

_____

_____

_____

signed _____
                                                                    Assistant

Actions Taken

☐ Chart marked and copy of problem form placed in chart.

☐ Information assembled for doctor's review.

☐ Patient notified of actions being taken.

Final Resolution

_____

_____

_____

_____

Date _____

●

Chapter 9

Low-Key Promotional Activities That Have an Impact on Patient Flow

Advertising, as distasteful as it may sound to some practitioners, is effective when it is properly and carefully executed. A marketing program can be very low key or very aggressive; the extent to which advertising is low key depends on the level of aggressiveness physicians are taking regarding promotion in your particular community. In some areas of the United States none of the physicians listed in the yellow pages have their names in bold face type, while in other communities, physicians may announce their services with quarter-page or half-page advertisements. In one community a very small box advertisement would be considered aggressive, while elsewhere the same approach would be though low key.

As a general rule in developing a marketing program, never be more aggressive in the promotion of your practice than you have to be. For example, if no physicians in the community have small box ads in the yellow pages, there is no real need for you to buy a quarter-page ad when a smaller, more "tasteful" ad will suffice. Before you plan your promotional activities, consider what the American Medical Association has to say about the ethics of it. The official position places no restrictions on advertising by physicians, except to protect the public from deceptive practices. The AMA's official position, as quoted from the *American Medical News*, January 23, 1981, is as follows:

There are no restrictions on advertising by physicians except those that can be specifically justified to protect the public from deceptive practices. A physician may publicize himself as a physician through any commercial publicity or other form of public communication (including any newspaper, magazine, telephone directory, radio, television or other advertising) provided that the communication shall not be misleading because of the omission of necessary material information, shall not contain any false or misleading statement, or shall not otherwise operate to deceive.

The form of communication should be designed to communicate the information contained therein to the public in a direct, dignified and readily comprehensive manner. Aggressive, high pressure advertising and publicity may create unjustified medical expectations. Any advertisement or publicity, regardless of format or content should be true and not misleading.

The communication may include: (a) the educational background of the physician; (b) the basis on which fees are determined (including charges for specific services); (c) available credit or other methods of payment; and (d) other information about the physician which a reasonable person might regard as relevant in determining whether to seek the physician's services.

Testimonials of patients, however, as to the physician's skill or the quality of his professional services should not be publicized. Statements relating to the quality of medical services are extremely difficult, if not impossible, to verify or measure by objective standards. Claims regarding experience, competence, and the quality of the physician's services may be made if they can be factually supported and if they do not imply that he has an exclusive and unique skill or remedy. A statement that a physician has cured or successfully treated a large number of cases involving a particular serious ailment may imply a certainty of result and create unjustified and misleading expectations in prospective patients.

Consistent with federal regulatory standards which apply to commercial advertising, a physician who is considering the placement of an advertisement or publicity release, whether in print, radio, or television, should determine in advance that his communication or message is explicitly and implicitly truthful and not misleading. These standards require the advertiser to have a reasonable basis for claims before they are used in advertising. The reasonable basis must be established by those facts known to the advertiser, and those which a reasonable, prudent advertiser should have discovered.

As used herein, reference to a "physician" applies also to information relating to the physician's group, partners, or associates. Any communication or message within the scope of the opinion should include the name of at least one physician responsible for its content.

My interpretation of these guidelines is that you can advertise or promote your services using any medium you deem appropriate with no restriction on size, presentation, and color. In the area of what you can say, however, the AMA is explicit. They do not want you to make statements as to the quality of your service that you cannot empirically back up, or make any statements whatsoever that could be interpreted as misleading. They specifically caution against the use of testimonials.

You should be aware that these are the AMA's national guidelines; you must also pay close attention to precedents and norms established within your own state and county. Each state and county interprets the guidelines differently. It is also important to consider what other physicians in your area are doing. It is unwise for a practitioner to deviate too far from the level of aggressiveness in your area.

Allocation of Advertising Budget

Consider the amount of money you have to spend to develop a tasteful program. You need to allow enough money to have high-quality, creative work and to advertise frequently enough.

Because the quality of an advertisement is important you should hire a commercial artist. While you could save money by allowing the newspaper to provide the layout for your advertisement, they usually offer stock art work and your promotion will look the same as those for pet and hardware stores. Since this is not the end effect you want to achieve, you must be prepared to spend the money to do it right. Creativity is also important. The advertisement should project the professional image of your practice without compromising your quality. You do not want to be gimmicky but you do want the display to stand out and be noticed.

If you are going to advertise, you have to do it boldly and with quality. One rule of print advertising is to try to dominate the page. This means that the size and boldness of your advertisement should be such that it attracts the most attention on that page. If there is little or no physician advertising in a particular publication and you have a small advertisement, obviously you will be dominating the page. However, in a newspaper or a local magazine that has advertising for your competition, you must be prepared to compete a little more aggressively with other messages. If you are conservative about your visibility, you should not consider advertising. On the other hand, if you decide to advertise, do it creatively and effectively, and try to capture the attention of the reader.

The frequency of your message has to be considered. There is no use placing an advertisement once, because that gives you little or no benefit. For an advertisement to be successful, it needs to be there over and over again. Frequency is very important in establishing your service in the minds of potential patients.

When you have carefully analyzed what your competition is doing, taken stock of your own promotional campaign, and laid out a reasonable budget, you will be ready to examine a variety of promotional mechanisms which will allow you to build your practice.

Remember, you should not be any more aggressive than you have to be. Promote tastefully, do it well, and be prepared to put the budget behind it. How much of a budget? It depends on your objectives, but you should consider somewhere between 5 and 15 percent of your gross income depending on the nature of competition in your area.

Types of Promotional Activities

Promotional activities that involve creation of patient rapport in the practice are especially useful. *Patient information booklets* (which are covered in detail later in this book) are an excellent way of dispensing information about the practice to prospective and established patients, and can be an ethical medical public relations tool.

Newsletters to your patients are another way of dispensing good medical advice. These newsletters are well read and stimulate interest, and they are also passed around to various physicians.

Sending Christmas cards and birthday cards to referral sources and patients is another public relations and promotional tool. As you can see, this approach may be a little more aggressive than the previous ones but it can be done very tastefully.

Write a regular weekly column on issues of medical interest. Many of the local newspapers read by patients in your drawing area are looking for columns. Many physicians who write such columns find that it is a good way of building a practice and that it gives them exposure and educates their patients. This is especially appropriate for physicians in one-newspaper towns.

Radio and television talk shows are included among the more aggressive strategies. Patients are always interested in topics of medical interest, and it is also a good way of building a practice. When using this and other of the more aggressive techniques, you should seek professional advice. You can do as much damage to your practice through blatant solicitation as you can to improve it, if your approach is not professional enough.

The yellow pages is a very effective place to advertise for new patients. A number of studies have indicated that many patients find their physicians through the yellow pages. This type of advertising can be expensive but it is an important source of practice growth. As mentioned earlier, you should never promote more aggressively than you need to—it depends on what your colleagues are doing. If your competitors are only listing their practices, for example, consider just putting your name in bold face type. If a number of other physicians have their names in bold face, you might then use a small box advertisement. If a number of physicians have small box advertisements, consider a quarter-page display. It's a good idea to be just a little more aggressive than your colleagues, so that your message can dominate the page.

As new types of health care delivery become available, we are beginning to see more *direct mail* sent to householders. A number of the large national physician groups are seeking patients through direct solicitation, using high-quality materials. Should you consider direct mail to householders, you will want to establish that you are mailing to a quality list. For example, a number of physicians buy lists from credit card companies because people have to be reasonably stable to be approved for credit privileges. In this way, you are promoting to the segment of the patient market that has already established good credit and will not be a potential credit liability to your practice.

There are many promotional activities that you can become involved in; choose them carefully and appropriately. A patient information booklet and a newsletter can be produced immediately. Writing a column in a newspaper is a conservative educational tool that might be good for some. Sending Christmas cards is also a tactful promotional medium.

When you consider direct mail advertising and yellow page advertising, you want to be sure that you are very careful to assess your local community standards and that your approach is right for you. When you have made your choices, make certain that the end result is a quality piece of work that is impeccably professional.

As medicine becomes more competitive, you will find that promotion will play an increasingly larger role in practice growth and development. Tastefully done and integrated in your practice enhancement program, these useful low-key techniques can affect your patient flow and practice growth.

●

Chapter 10

Patient Satisfaction: The Key to Practice Success

Every successful practice has a large base of happy, satisfied patients who spread the good word about their physician to others. Achieving patient satisfaction with your practice involves more than merely meeting your patients' medical service needs. You need to focus on improving your augmented service in the areas of financial arrangements and other areas that are not specifically related to the delivery of care. It is important to assure yourself that patients are happy not only with the service they receive from you personally, but also with your practice systems and procedures, staff, and other amenities.

Patients seek not only a physician who is qualified medically, but also a practice that provides personalized service. To deliver personalized service you must understand your patients and what they expect from your practice. This is the essence of practice enhancement.

Understanding Patient Satisfaction Issues

If you can, try to determine the average age of your patients and the predominant demographic characteristics of the entire practice.

Although it may seem fairly obvious to you at first, you may be surprised at the results.

Your objective is to develop a clear profile of the average patient in your practice. While each patient is, of course, unique, you will probably be able to make some generalizations about them. For example, you would have to structure the systems, procedures, and appointment scheduling in a different manner if the average age of your patients was 65 than you would if the average age was about 30. If you have a number of families with small children, you will want to include a children's play section in your reception area. You might also consider having supervised baby-sitting at certain peak times. You will also need to know where your patients live. In a primary care practice, patients should live no more than 20 minutes from your practice. If you have patients who live farther than this, you might consider moving your practice to a more central location.

Keep abreast of your neighborhood and its changes. One internist in California had a patient base that changed over the years to one of a significantly older population as his middle-aged executives moved away. His practice received a tremendous boost when he began calling it a geriatric clinic, signifying this new practice focus. He restructured his systems and procedures to fit his older population.

Patient satisfaction is elusive and ever changing. Practitioners who understand their patients' demographic characteristics are better able to understand what satisfies them and to change along with them.

Find Out What Your Patients Really Think of Your Practice

The best way to determine how to keep your patients satisfied is to ask them their opinions. It is a good idea to survey them routinely, and ask them how you can improve your service to them. They'll tell you. Use the practice evaluation card, which you can send directly to the patient, as mentioned in the previous chapter.

Another way to obtain good information about your patients' current level of satisfaction is to get them more directly involved in the management of your practice. Some practitioners have set up practice advisory committees (in market research terms, we call these *focus groups;* in a focus group, the market researcher randomly selects a number of patients from a particular community and surveys them with key questions about the service). In your focus group or patient advisory council you will preselect your patients and meet with them at least on a monthly basis to obtain feedback on how you might develop your practice and keep your patients better satisfied. The information gathered from these sessions is invaluable. One physician has different patients from his practice in the group each month, with the goal of involving each of his patients in at least one meeting.

Understanding why patients leave your practice gives you excellent insight into patient satisfaction with your practice. I know one doctor who calls all patients who have left his practice and conducts an "exit interview"—even for those who have relocated. Patients who are leaving and feel their relationship with you is terminated will give you more frank feedback than they would if they felt they would be with you for a number of years. It is useful to ask specifically whether the patient left because he or she was dissatisfied with the service. More often than not you will find that the departure was the result of some policy that you could change, or due to a staff member's attitude, which also could be changed.

A good research base will give you a great deal of information on how to keep your patients satisfied. Patient satisfaction stems from all elements of your practice, beginning with a high-quality service. It starts with the first telephone call and continues through the last payment of the bill. Everything should be professional and patient centered. Focus on practice efficiency should be secondary to patient wants. There is always a way of working out a new system to ensure a high level of patient satisfaction.

Your Staff

Your success, your patients' satisfaction, and your ability to compete in the marketplace are more directly influenced by your staff than by any other element of practice enhancement. Warm, friendly, and helpful staff members with a positive approach to working will help form the foundation for a thriving and growing practice; they are truly the ambassadors of your practice, and they have that all-important first contact with your patients.

As you are aware, creating the ideal team of ambassadors takes time and effort. You are aiming to develop a delicate balance between patient satisfaction through high staff morale and motivation and the production of high-quality work. Chapter 15 lays out a system for recruitment to help you in this area.

Four basic building blocks—(1) the use of specific job descriptions, (2) an effective organization, (3) performance appraisals, and (4) written personnel policies—form the foundation for a successful personnel management program as part of enhancing your practice. With them you will be able to manage your staff effectively.

To achieve an *effective organization,* you must ensure that staff members know who their boss is and what their responsibilities are to each of their co-workers. A clear organizational chart of the practice should be prepared. Chapter 11 outlines several ways of addressing this issue.

The development of *specific job descriptions* for each staff member requires that you know what you expect to be done and the level of expertise required; it is important to commit this to paper. Your job description becomes a key element in the recruiting, hiring, training, and motivational process of the practice. Chapter 12 discusses specific aspects of how to develop job descriptions.

Performance appraisals are another important aspect of an effective patient-oriented team. The job descriptions state specifically what needs to be accomplished, while performance appraisals lay out standards of how the job is to be completed successfully. Staff members require ongoing feedback about how well they are completing their jobs and whether they are meeting your required level of performance. Chapter 13 shows you how to implement a system of performance appraisals in your practice.

Written personnel policies state the rules and regulations that are required in an effectively run operation. They cover such items as working hours, sick pay, vacation, and grounds for dismissal. They can range from a two-page written document in an individual practice to a multi-page document in a group. Chapter 14 deals with personnel policies, and Chapter 16 deals with the termination process. Your staff projects some important images to your patients; you must ensure that it is the image which you want you patients to absorb, and thus you must help staff members understand and foster your attitudes and feelings toward your patients.

Once you have developed and implemented the four key building blocks to an effective personnel management program, you will have the basis for running your practice for the benefit of your patients, with a satisfied, team-oriented staff at your side. Because your staff are the envoys of your medical practice philosophy, it is critical that you invest time and effort to ensure that they are managed properly in performing their duties at the high levels that you and your patients deserve.

It is not my intent to discriminate against male medical assistants and nurses; however, for ease of use and personalization this section refers to staff members in the female gender.

Chapter 11

Organizing Your Practice for Patient Satisfaction and Practice Success

The most successful practices, like the most successful businesses, are well-organized units that clearly understand their direction and goals. Successful practices are in the business of helping people, and the goal is not only treating patients but also keeping them satisfied. To do this we must be organized and able to delegate responsibility, to ensure that the goals of the practice are being met.

A clear-cut organizational system must be established in a medical practice to enable it to compete and to deliver quality care to patients effectively. Once the system is implemented, you will find that your practice is able to achieve maximum productivity and to facilitate communication among you, your staff, and your patients, in a friction-free environment. Good organization helps you clarify what needs to be done and helps you manage your practice in an easy, effective manner.

One dictionary defines *organize* as the way to "arrange or constitute in interdependent parts, each having a special function or relation with respect to the whole." Your job will be to lay out a framework to ensure that a complex number of systems, procedures, and people are organized to deliver the standard of service or care to your patients, always remembering that the overall goal and perspective of the practice is to keep the patient satisfied.

Isolate the Key Variables to Practice Success

From a service perspective, a medical practice has three clearly defined areas—(1) patient relations, (2) clinical interaction, and (3) financial and administrative organization—where the practice interacts with the patient to deliver the service. Each area is interdependent with the others, and how well each area is managed affects overall patient satisfaction and practice profitability.

Patient relations is the area of the practice that deals with the ongoing communication of the practice with the patient and outside people; typically, this role is taken by the receptionist. Practice success and failure can be directly correlated to how well your practice relates with the patients. The receptionist usually has more contact with the patient than do other staff members; however, nurses and aides (and you yourself) spend significant time relating with patients. These interactions create an impression that has little to do with the actual clinical service or financial matters. This area of patient relations is primary in a successful medical practice.

Clinical interaction relates to the aspect of the practice that is organized to deliver care to the patients. It begins with the prehistory form that the patient needs to fill out, followed by the initial screening by the nurse, your clinical evaluation and diagnosis, and the actual medical care. This is the area of the practice on which most physicians and staff focus. Obviously, the quality of the service that patients receive is directly related to how well your practice is organized to deliver the clinical aspect of the practice.

Financial and administrative organization relates specifically to a smooth patient visit. Typically, this area involves credit and collection policies, policies requiring payment at the time of service, production of typed reports, and all of those systems and procedures that assist in the overall standard of practice efficiency and profitability.

In developing each of these three areas of practice, you must remember what you are working toward—keeping the customer satisfied. It is the areas of patient relations, clinical administration, and financial coordination that truly differentiate a successful practice from one that is just getting by.

Figure **11-1.** Medical practice organizational structure for an individual practice that is just starting up.

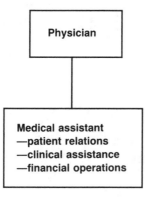

Post Your Organizational Chart

Staff members need to know specifically what their responsibilities are. To clearly delineate this, it is important that you develop an organizational chart, which should clearly establish who is in charge, to whom they are responsible, and what their specific areas of responsibilities are.

Figure 11-1 is an example of a physician with one medical assistant who performs three basic types of duties—patient relations, clinical coordination, and financial matters. The physician with only one staff member also overlaps in those three areas, as he or she may go out and get the patients, fill out a number of the clinical forms, and get involved with some of the financial details of the practice.

As the practice expands, it will move into an organizational unit such as seen in Figure 11-2, where the physician may have three staff members; the primary responsibility of the receptionist is patient relations. The clinical area would typically be the responsibility of the nurse, and the third area would fall to a financial coordinator or bookkeeper.

Figure 11-3 shows a larger clinical organization; we now have a patient relations department, which is typically the reception and front desk area of the practice. It may be subdivided into the following categories: reception, telephone answering, appointment making, and patient records management, as well as responsibility for new patients. At this level there would be clinical and financial departments; each department should be headed by a supervisor.

The development of an organizational chart allows everyone to know

Figure **11-2.** Medical practice organizational structure for an established individual practice.

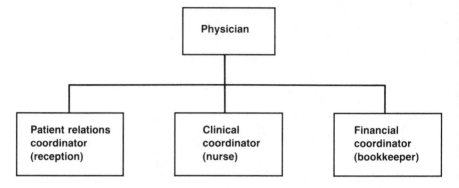

specifically to whom they are responsible; this helps you to control the key variables for success in an organized and well-thought-out manner.

People Can Only Relate to One Boss

In any successful organization, staff members can relate to only one person as their boss. In a one-staff-person office, this is relatively simple to do, since there is only one person responsible. However, you should clearly delineate the role of your spouse in the practice, as well as the role of your accountant and the responsibilities of your medical assistant. Your office staff members may be responsible for delivering some materials to those individuals but you are their boss.

Organizational conflicts over who is boss become more evident when you get into a three-person office. Typically, the medical assistant who has been there the longest begins to exert some control over the other members of the group. An organizational chart clearly delineates that the physician is still in charge. Resist the temptation to abdicate your responsibility as the boss, unless you are prepared to designate one person as supervisor of the total group. Sometimes it is valuable for a practice to designate a supervisor as soon as there are more than two people in the practice. However, should you do this, you need to post the organizational chart and be prepared to delegate the responsibility to the applicable person.

Describe the Positions Creatively

In a patient-centered practice, patients spend more time relating with your staff members than they do with you. Normally, we use lowly titles

Figure 11-3. Medical practice organizational structure for a group practice staff.

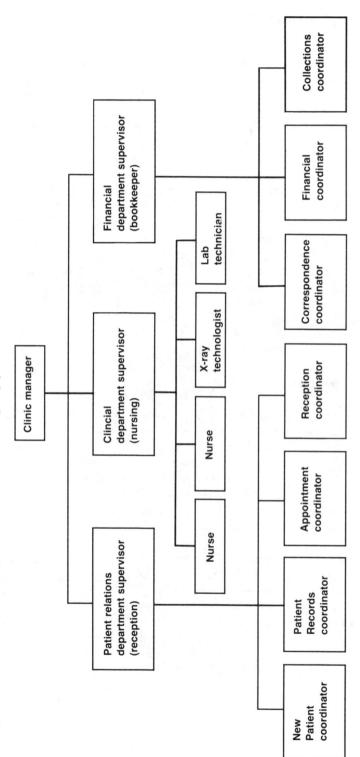

for staff members, such as bookkeeper or file clerk; however, I strongly recommend that you use the title of patient relations coordinator instead of receptionist, clinical coordinator rather than nurse, and financial coordinator in preference to bookkeeper. These are two positive effects for the practice. First, patients will relate better to a person with a positive and important-sounding title; second, your staff will have a higher sense of self-worth if the title clearly reflects the level of responsibility.

One physician gave the title of communications coordinator to the file clerk. This had an astounding impact upon the file clerk, as she was now responsible for all of the inner office and patient communication items so that she would know where they were. This transformed the less meaningful job of storing paper in files to a more important level; the clerk now began to view the job as not only one that involved knowing where the paper was, but also one that included devising systems and procedures for the clinic to ensure that communications were well laid out in the practice. (Besides, if you were at a party, which would you rather say you were—communications coordinator for Dr. Jones's office or file clerk?)

Retain Your Leadership

Since managing the practice demands much attention, it is easy to abdicate the responsibility of leadership and devote all your attention to the full-time clinical aspects of the practice. When physicians abdicate their leadership responsibility, however, the resulting deterioration of staff morale and patient service has been reflected in unsuccessful practices. Your staff need to be motivated, led, and evaluated, to ensure that the goals of your organization are being met, and this requires your leadership and time.

You have to ensure that the patients' needs are being met, that your staff members are well directed, and that the goals of your practice are clearly laid out. Successful practices are established and maintained by physicians who can achieve a sense of perspective about the need for satisfying the customer and the importance of a good organizational structure. Organization is key to an efficient, effective practice enhancement program. Patient relations, clinical organization, and financial administrative organization must work together to deliver the highest level of care and service to patients.

———————————————————————————————●

Chapter 12

Patient-Centered Job Descriptions

All the tasks that seem mechanical—putting files away, sending out collection letters, and all the paper work—are done with the goal of helping the patient. A successful medical practice is in the business of satisfying patients' wants and desires. The jobs are carried out to ensure the visit is as smooth, efficient, and pleasant as possible.

All staff members should be closely attuned to the needs of the patients. They should be aware that their primary responsibility, no matter what they are doing, is to the patient. Filling out that form, therefore, is far less important than meeting the needs of the patient standing at the window. Patient-centered job descriptions help us keep sight of what we are doing and why we are doing it. They relate what is being done in the practice to keeping the patients happy.

Why You Need Job Descriptions

Patient-centered job descriptions help us focus on what actually has to be done. They also assist us in the hiring process, since once we know what has to be done we have a good idea of the qualities, experience, and skills that the ideal candidate will have to possess.

Figure **12-1**

Job Qualifications:
Administrative medical assistant.

Education:
Prefer candidate with post-high-school secretarial and/or business training.

Skills:
1. Accurate typing of not less than 45 words per minute required.
2. Knowledge of basic bookkeeping procedures required.
3. Familiarity with insurance forms required.
4. Knowledge of medical terminology preferred.

Since job descriptions specifically describe the nature of the position and the responsibilities to the patient, they serve as an orientation to applicants and reminders to existing employees of what is expected of them. If an employee needs improvement in performance, a written job description will help her readjust her priorities. The job description acts as an aid to ensure that what ought to be done is being done, always keeping the needs of the patient primary. Figure 12-1 is an example of a job qualification sheet.

Job descriptions also assist in the termination process, because you can clearly point to the specific areas where performance is expected but is not being carried out. By breaking the job down into its logical components, you will be able to plan time frames and to assess whether you are overstaffed.

Implementing Job Descriptions

Before you can design an accurate, detailed job description, you should perform a job analysis, which will enable you to break down all the tasks and duties that need to be carried out and to estimate how long each should take. This can be done with a minimum amount of disruption in your office if you use current staff members to do it. You should encourage your staff to engage in brainstorming and write down every task that they do—for example, opening the office, turning on the lights, taking the covers off the equipment, turning the coffee machine on, setting up a new Day Sheet, opening the appointment book, taking the cash out of the safe and placing it in the cash drawer, and reviewing the In Box today to see what has to be done. An office time standards development sheet (as shown in Figure 12-2) can be used for making this list of all the tasks that each job entails. The time estimates can be handled later.

Get Maximum Staff Involvement

The staff members will realize the importance of their jobs and job descriptions if you gain their cooperation as a part of the process and procedure. Job descriptions should be introduced as a positive benefit to the staff, since the process will assist them in clearly delineating what needs to be done. Staff members will know what tasks have to be performed and how long these will take. I would suggest giving each one a form on which they can itemize each job as it is completed. They can also determine the average time each takes.

As each task is done, the staff member should relate it to the benefit it extends to the patients. For instance, when the patient's chart is obtained ahead of time, the assistant should be aware that this helps ensure a more successful patient/doctor visit. Even the most ordinary task, such as filing, can be related back as a patient benefit.

Notice on Figure 12-2 that there is a place for how long tasks take— with your estimate and your staff's estimate as well as the actual time used. You may only want to time them when the estimates differ. You may also want to add any tasks that have been omitted, or any that you feel are now required.

If you are a new physician starting up practice, read the current literature and construct your job analysis to the best of your ability before you open. Do it while you have the time! You can rework the descriptions quickly three months later, when you have more experience behind you.

Patient-Centered Job Titles

A job title can create a positive impact not only on your patients but also on your staff, by improving morale. For example, consider the title of patient-relations coordinator, rather than receptionist. This is patient centered and has a nice ring to it. I like using the word coordinator wherever I can; collections coordinator sounds better than collections clerk. Other possibilities are information coordinator instead of file clerk, and clinical care coordinator in place of nurse.

Titles do not cost you more, but they can provide a tangible benefit to your staff and have a positively effect on you and your patients.

Figure **12-2**

Task	Benefit to patient	Monday			Tuesday		
		Your estimate	Staff's estimate	Actual	Your estimate	Staff's estimate	Actual
1							
2							
3							
4							
5							
6							
7							
8							
9							
10							
11							
12							
13							
14							

Wednesday			Thursday			Friday		
Your estimate	Staff's estimate	Actual	Your estimate	Staff's estimate	Actual	Your estimate	Staff's estimate	Actual

Therefore, after you agree on the title, the next step is to lay out a summary of the position; the following is an example of one such summary:

Position summary: Patient relations coordinator

Responsible for creating the first positive impression with patients on the telephone and in person, as well as for handling all the necessary forms and paper work to ensure a pleasant and positive experience at the office.

Maintains the general appearance and cleanliness of the examination rooms and business and reception areas, to create a pleasing first impression.

Answers all incoming telephone calls in such a way as to discern and satisfy patient needs.

Grouping Tasks Into Duty Blocks

From your brainstorm sheet of tasks (see Figure 12-2), you should group specific tasks into duty blocks, which summarizes a group of related tasks. One duty block would be: "Handles all incoming telephone calls." A patient-centered duty block tells what generally has to be done and why; one example would be: "Answers all incoming telephone calls in order to discern and satisfy the needs of the patient." Another example of a duty block is: "Interviews patients and explains the proper method of handling and preparing insurance claims in order to ensure timely payment from the insurance company to the patient or practice." The duty is always written in the present tense and begins with a specific action verb.

It is also important to include the reason why the duty should be performed. Take this opportunity to reinforce the importance of every duty in terms of satisfying the needs of your patients. This emphasis becomes clear in the example: "Maintains the general appearance and cleanliness of the examination rooms in order to give patients a feeling of confidence that their services are being met in a well-kept facility."

Each duty block consists of several related tasks. These tasks tell how the duty is to be performed. Figure 12-3 is an example of a duty block—the left column denotes the duty, which tells generally what is to be done, and why; the middle column lists all the tasks involved in that duty; and the right column estimates the average amount of time allotted for each duty.

Figure **12-3.** Duty block describing tasks involved in handling incoming telephone calls.

Duty	Tasks	Time
Answers all incoming telephone calls	Answers within 3 rings Identifies the office by use of doctor's name—e.g., "Dr. Smith's office" Identifies herself by her own name—e.g., "Sally speaking." Offers assistance: "May I help you?" Gives the reason why doctor can't come to the phone immediately Asks the caller's name early in the conversation and uses it Tells when the call will be returned Asks if the caller minds being on hold, and then wait for a response Follows each call to its logical conclusion Speaks in a pleasant, courteous tone with a clear distinct voice Maintains a positive attitude and a helpful approach	1–2 minutes per call on average

State the Supervision to Be Received

Briefly describe why it is important to state clearly to whom the person is responsible. It avoids misunderstandings when staff members know who their boss is, who will give them directions, and who will evaluate them, as well as who will help them in problem solving.

It is understandable that confusion can occur when the line of authority is unclear. A medical assistant in a one-doctor office, for example, receives directions from many different people, including the physician, the accountant, the physician's spouse, and others. Many times, although the medical assistant may report to the doctor, someone else may be specifically responsible for hiring, training, and firing her. The direction of responsibility should be made clear. It is also important to let the staff member know what people they must coordinate with and what their responsibilities are to the other persons in the office.

Obviously, there is an overlap on all tasks in a physician's practice. It is critical to establish this specifically at the outset. For example, the medical assistant may have to coordinate with the accountant or the doctor's spouse; in a larger practice, the medical assistant may be responsible to a supervisor and will have to coordinate with the nurse and the bookkeeper.

Sign the Job Descriptions

By signing their job descriptions, new employees are confirming that they have read, understood, and agreed to the duties and tasks that they must perform. This confirmation is an agreement saying they understand to whom they are responsible and with whom they are expected to coordinate; this procedure influences their commitment to the job. It is also essential to include the date of the signature, in case legal problems should arise in the future, if the employee is fired.

Qualifications for the Ideal Employee

Job descriptions assist you in the hiring process by giving you a clear picture of the ideal person to perform the job. A separate sheet for job qualifications should include experience, education, and skills that are important if the job is to be performed well. A job description helps you visualize the type of person you want when you advertise the position. By knowing what you are looking for, you can easily communicate it in an advertisement.

A typical job description might show that to qualify for the position a person needs a high school diploma or (preferably) a secretarial school diploma, two years experience in a medical office, the ability to type 65 words per minute, knowledge of basic bookkeeping procedures, and familiarity with insurance forms.

Job descriptions are critical in the orientation of a new staff member, since they clearly delineate the responsibilities to the physician, and, most important, the responsibilities to the patients. In the orientation process, it is important to highlight the fact that the job is to keep the patient satisfied and to explain how all the tasks relate to this.

Figure **12-4.** Patient-centered job description. The duty blocks are filled in as shown in Figure 12-3.

Job Title: General medical assistant/receptionist

Position summary: Responsible for all the general administration, clinical assistance
   and financial aspects of the practice

Supervision received: directly responsible to Dr. Smith; liason with Mr. Jones, Dr.
   Smith's accountant, and Mrs. Smith

	Duty Blocks	
Duty	**Task Related**	**Time**
(1) . . .		
(2) . . .		
(3) . . .		

Employee's Signature _____ Date _____

Figure 12-4 is a sample of how a patient-centered medical office job description may look when the job title, position summary and duty blocks, supervision received and signature date correspond to a well-coordinated form.

Your patients are your most valuable assets to the practice. Everyone in the practice should work to protect and promote those assets. Patient-centered duty blocks ensure that the best possible job is being done to help the patients. The focus of a patient-centered job description is less on the tasks and more on the reasons why the job exists—and that's to keep the patients satisfied.

Chapter 13

Rating Your Staff's Performance: Keeping the Personnel Edge

Can you guarantee quality service to your patients in every encounter? Warranties and guarantees are well established in product purchases; however, they are more elusive and harder to ensure in the service sector. The closest thing to a guarantee of service in a medical practice is the implementation of regular performance appraisals. These quality control measures increase your office efficiency, productivity, and cost-effectiveness, and they influence patient well-being and represent an integrated mechanism in your practice enhancement program.

A performance appraisal is a method for judging how well your staff members are executing their jobs. To judge quality, it is critical to form a specific definition for an expected standard of performance. The performance appraisal compares the performance of your staff member with that level.

Benefits of Performance Appraisals

Performance appraisals open valuable and informative communication lines between you and your staff. For example, in discussing appointment scheduling problems, you may feel your assistant is poor at booking. During the dialogue you may discover what the problem really is and begin to develop a solution; you may find out that it is actually you who are throwing off the schedule.

Performance appraisals also help you clarify exactly what is to be done and determine the relative importance of tasks that are not performed satisfactorily, as well as define the level of performance that you expect. Your staff is much more likely to perform better when they understand exactly what is expected of them.

You can, in addition, use performance appraisals as an opportunity to compliment your staff for work well done (we all need praise and encouragement to motivate us to do better). When work continues to be unsatisfactory, performance appraisals assist us in the termination process. Only when we can specifically uncover why staff members are not performing can we move to do something about it.

Basic Considerations

The evaluation process has two components: (1) a daily judging process involving frequent monitoring of staff members' work, and (2) a formal appraisal, which ought to be done for 30 minutes twice a year.

You should regard the performance appraisal not just as a good or bad report card but rather as an opportunity to improve your staff's performance. Time invested in feedback (both positive and negative) regarding your staff's work and in making concrete plans for improvement will pay you dividends in the long run.

Establish the Criteria for Performance.

Before you design your performance appraisal format, consider how your staff will measure up. Think about the following: (1) the affective (attitudinal) and cognitive criteria that you used when you hired this person, (2) the written job description agreed upon on hiring, and (3) your current ideas of what constitutes good medical office management. Then, compile this list, along with such pertinent information as name, job title, date hired, and so forth, on the appraisal form.

Figure 13-1 is a sample of a medical assistant's performance appraisal. It is especially applicable in the office of an individual practitioner. For this purpose, the form has been divided into three sections. Section A

Figure 13-1

Patient-Centered Performance Evaluation Form

Name _____
Position _____
Date of last review _____
Date of hiring _____
Review period _____
Type of review: (a) Probationary _____ (b) Annual _____ (c) Other (specify) _____

Section A
Job Skills

	Rating		
	Improvmt. Needed	**Standard**	**Above Standard**
(1) Patient rapport/relations Has high level of rapport and respect from patients as witnessed by positive patient feedback and/or personal observations.	☐	☐	☐
Comment: _____			
(2) Job knowledge Thoroughly familiar with how to execute all aspects of job.	☐	☐	☐
Comment: _____			
(3) Job execution Able to complete all aspects of job with a high degree of excellence, in a timely manner.	☐	☐	☐
Comment: _____			
(4) Organization and ability to plan Anticipates problems. Works and plans job effectively and efficiently. (Does everything have its place?)	☐	☐	☐
Comment: _____			
(5) Cost and efficiency orientation Judiciously utilizes staff time, equipment, and supplies to maximize output. (Biggest factor is good use of staff time.)	☐	☐	☐
Comment: _____			
(6) Maximizes doctor's time Suggests and implements methods to reduce physician involvement in nonmedical or routine tasks.	☐	☐	☐
Comment: _____			

Section B
Attitudes

Rating

	Improvmt. Needed	Standard	Above Average
(1) Patient orientation Truly believes the "customer is king" and patients' needs come first.	☐	☐	☐
Comment: _____			
(2) Positive attitude Displays a positive demenor toward patients, co-workers, doctor, and work.	☐	☐	☐
Comment: _____			
(3) Cooperation Works cooperatively with doctor and other team members.	☐	☐	☐
Comment: _____			
(4) Initiative Suggests improvements and implements new ideas without directives to do so where necessary.	☐	☐	☐
Comment: _____			
(5) Judgment Displays good judgment in problem solving.	☐	☐	☐
Comment: _____			
(6) Reliability Accepts responsibility and can be relied on to complete duties in timely manner.	☐	☐	☐

Comment: _____

Section C
Personal Attributes

	Rating		
	Improvmt. Needed	Standard	Above Standard
(1) People oriented/outgoing Generally likes people and prefers to be with them and work with them (patient skill, good attitude about people)	☐	☐	☐
Comment: _____			
(2) Production oriented Focuses on producing large amounts of work at a fast rate.	☐	☐	☐
Comment: _____			
(3) Quality oriented Focuses on completing work with high degree of accuracy and excellence.	☐	☐	☐
Comment: _____			
(4) Performance under pressure Is able to perform well under pressure.	☐	☐	☐
Comment: _____			
(5) Ability to work unsupervised Works well without supervision or direction.	☐	☐	☐
Comment: _____			
(6) Appearance Is always presentable, neat, and attractive.	☐	☐	☐
Comment: _____			
(7) Punctuality and attendance Always starts and ends on time. Is rarely absent without good reason.	☐	☐	☐

Comment: _____

deals with the cognitive realm of job skills. These are all easily measured because they are more concrete. One area that falls into the job-skills designation is excellent patient relations. Performance here can be determined by your observations, as well as through feedback from patients—both verbal and on formal feedback forms.

Format of Performance Appraisal

Job Skills

In terms of job skills, knowledge of the job is critical. Job knowledge refers to understanding the nature of the job, knowing how to perform all the required duties, and being familiar with all the machinery related to that job.

Job execution requires that the tasks be completed accurately and on time—essential requirements in the job skills area. You can determine the quality of performance by referring to the job description that your assistant signed during the hiring period. In fact, it would speed up the process if you were to clip the job description to this part of the appraisal form.

Analysis of job skills relates specifically to the job description. Efficiency is a must if your practice is to be competitive in today's market. This factor is dealt with in terms of the medical assitant's personal organization and ability to plan, her orientation for the relationship between cost and efficiency, and her ability to maximize your time and make you more efficient.

Organization and ability to plan refer to your medical assistant's ability to anticipate problems and set priorities in planning her day's work and carry out those tasks efficiently. As you evaluate in this area, you might ask yourself: "Does she anticipate that I will be running late, and take appropriate measures, such as calling to let patients know— or rescheduling them?"

The cost and efficiency factor evaluates whether your aide can coordinate the use of her time with equipment and supplies, to maximize her output. For example, does she use the backs of outdated forms for scrap paper, or does she order special paper for such purposes?

As critical as your assistant's own efficiency is her capability to maximize your time. She can do this by helping you reduce your involvement in routine, nonmedical tasks. These efficiency issues are determined by your daily observation. For example, does she support your dictating the information for your charts, as opposed to your writing it in yourself? It is with her support that systems and procedures can be implemented to help you function at your highest level.

Attitudes

Section B of the performance appraisal is more subjective, as it deals with the area of attitudes. Although they are more difficult to evaluate because they are based on judgment, they are just as critical to the success of your practice. Good attitudes foster good public relations and good productivity, in a pleasant working environment. Six attitudes in particular are key if your practice is to stay competitive.

1. Your medical assistants must possess a *patient orientation*. They must have a deep understanding and appreciation for the philosophy, "the customer is king," and be cognizant of the fact that, without patients, there would be no job for your medical assistant. One way in which she will have demonstrated this orientation is in taking a problem-solving approach to handling hostile patient problems in collections. The technique is to educate the patient to understand the problem; however, the assistant should always be aware of the possibility that she could be wrong and the patient right.

2. An assistant who displays a *positive attitude* toward patients, co-workers, and other employees makes the office a pleasant place for everyone. Patients appreciate the friendly atmosphere of an office in which everyone tries to behave pleasantly and professionally. The assistant will have demonstrated this attitude by being cheerful and friendly, even when patients are backed up in the office and it is an unusually hectic day; also she will usually not criticize others behind their backs for making errors, but will address ways to correct those errors.

3. In order for you and the other members of your staff to be truly effective, there must be a spirit of cooperation among you. Your aides must understand and demonstrate *cooperation* in working with you and other members of your team, to enable delivery of the best possible health care to your patients. One of the ways in which she might do this is to work as a team member to ensure that billing information is cross-checked by both the nurses and the front desk.

4. Since your assistant is the closest person to the clerical side of your practice, she is more likely to see better ways of getting different tasks done. It is important, therefore, that she be able to

take the *initiative* in making appropriate clerical improvements, without explicit directions from you. For instance, if she sees a new form that will improve efficiency, she determines the prices, gets your approval, and implements the form without your prodding.

5. Because most medical assistants have such a variety of tasks to perform, many of which involve dealing with people, it is critical that your aide exercise *good judgment* in handling problems and priorities. This is particularly true of the sole practitioner's assistant whose judgments are an integral part of each day. The judgments made in dealing with such problems as overdue accounts, emergency patients, or appointment scheduling will affect your practice growth. Obviously then you can not afford to have an aide with poor judgment.

6. Since your time and energies are so drained with the direct responsibilities of patient care, it is absolutely essential to your peace of mind and productivity that you can rely on a medical assistant who can, and will, accept other responsibilities. You must be able to count on her *reliability* in accepting responsibility for completing all duties in an accurate and timely manner. Remember, she is there to help you—not the reverse. A medical assistant who is reliable will work late when required and authorized, to ensure that work is done and that the next day's operation is smooth.

Personal Attributes

The final section of the performance appraisal addresses the evaluation of personal attributes and traits that combine to produce a desirable and successful medical assistant. Ideally, we would be able to determine these during the interviewing process; however, our perceptions do change after we have worked with someone. This is the most subjective and therefore the most difficult part of the evaluation. Nevertheless, it is important to complete it, because it helps you focus on those areas of her personality that are basic to a good working relationship and on her ability to fulfill the rest of her duties.

The first three personal attributes critical to a successful medical assistant fall into the realm of public relations and personal dynamics. She must be *people oriented*. Generally speaking, she has more than just good skill when dealing with patients—she prefers to work with people. An aide who would prefer to be with others rather than to read in quiet seclusion is more likely to enhance practice growth.

It is equally important, though, that the medical assistant be *production oriented.* Because of the busy nature of the job, she must be able to focus on producing large amounts of work at a quick rate. Naturally, quality work must go hand-in-hand with efficient production. Your aide must be able to produce work with a high degree of quality and excellence. In addition, she should always find something to do during slack periods in the office, or when the doctor is not in. This work should also show a high level of quality because the person is intrinsically motivated to do a good job.

Since the individual practitioner's office is often a maze of ringing telephones, crowded waiting rooms, and stacks of invoices—all to be attended to in the same afternoon—it is vital that your medical assistant be able to *perform effectively under pressure* and to work *unsupervised* and undirected by you or another staff member. Ask yourself: "Is her performance hampered when she has three patients on the telephone, two waiting to be checked in, and two others waiting to pay their bills?"

Patients respect and appreciate a neat, clean office environment. You and your staff are the most important part of that environment. Therefore, *good personal grooming* is absolutely essential for staff members, in order to project a caring, professional image. Patients reason that any staff member who does not care enough to look her best has little concern about caring for others. Also, in an image-oriented competitive environment there is never a second chance for a first impression.

In a well-run practice, careful attention is given to scheduling. In order for schedules to run smoothly and deadlines to be met, it is important that your aide demonstrate a high regard for *punctuality* and *attendance.* If she is not at her desk at precisely opening time to answer the first telephone call, or if she is frequently absent and you have the inconvenience of finding a substitute to handle her work, she is disrupting the smooth operation of your practice and lowering the quality of services provided to patients.

The sample appraisal form should be adapted to your needs. Where possible, you should make the form as specific to your own specialty and practice as possible. Some of your ideal characteristics will differ. The job you're evaluating may involve many aspects; however, if you look at the three areas of job skill, attitudes, and personal attributes, they all help to make a truly successful medical assistant who is a valuable asset to your practice. Give a copy of your appraisal form to your medical assistant prior to the day of the interview. Ask her to fill it out privately, and bring it along to the interview. It will serve as a starting point for your discussions.

Appraisal Interview

Set Up the Right Conditions for a Performance Appraisal

Hold the appraisal interview in a private office where you are out of earshot of other employees and can speak openly. Also, free yourself from interruptions to avoid wasting your time, your train of thought, and your rapport with the staff member being evaluated.

Bring a Positive Attitude to the Appraisal

If you come to the interview thinking that all employees are just out to do as little as possible and collect as high a salary as possible, it will be difficult for you to develop the atmosphere for positive change. If you come to the interview feeling that there is no way that this person can change, chances are you will be right. You are most likely to get the best results if you regard the evaluation as an opportunity to help the staff member better understand how she can be more effective and feel more successful as an integral part of your team.

Conduct of the Interview

Since people are usually tense about evaluations, you should begin the interview with some techniques for setting the person at ease. Do this by letting her know you are interested in her as an individual. Ask about her family, her hobbies, and how things are going outside of the job. Let her know that you appreciate her contribution to the practice. You might say: "Sally, I want you to know how much I appreciate your professional handling of all patients." A simple remark like this will encourage continued high performance. Show that you want to help the staff member be as successful as possible. You can accomplish this by saying: "The focus of our discussion will be on how to develop you to the highest level of excellence you are capable of achieving."

Although both of you have completed your evaluations forms, focus on hers for discussion. Remember, it's her form that is going to be most important, since self-evaluation and change will be the key to her continued improvement. Dwell on the positives during the interview, and give recognition where it is due. Discuss those factors where your evaluations differ. In particular, talk in detail about those areas that need improvement. During this part of the discussion it is essential that you clarify the nature of the task that needs improvement, as well as its relative importance.

It is important to specify the level of performance and execution you expect on all tasks that have not heretofore been performed to your satisfaction. Lay out a specific plan of action toward improving the problem, and set down the expected end results and timetable for improvement in writing. Thus you might have: "Sally will have completely mastered the process of writing up Day Sheets by Thursday, August 30, as witnessed by five consecutive days without errors."

At the conclusion of the discussion, have your medical assistant sign the evaluation form. Not only does this impress on the staff member the seriousness of her commitment to your practice and the importance of your common objectives, it also serves as legal documentation should you ever need to fire her.

Having staff members who consistently perform effectively is essential to a successful practice. When performance appraisals are conducted and followed up professionally and regularly, they become key instruments in monitoring and improving your employees' level of performance, which helps keep your patients satisfied and aids your overall practice enhancement program.

Chapter 14

Personnel Policies That Keep Your Staff on Track

Practice Benefits of Personnel Policies

Motivated, productive staff members have a positive effect on practice growth because they focus on the patient's well being. Patients sense this and are more likely to refer their friends to you. The most difficult aspect of keeping your assistants productive involves the establishment of personnel policies—the "rules and regulations" that govern the staff's working conditions and the relationship between staff and physician. Every practice has such policies but few commit them to paper. As a result, personnel become disgruntled when the physician makes different or inconsistent rulings for individual staff members. In an effective practice enhancement system, written personnel policies are a necessity; this approach will circumvent many employee problems, as well as curtail much frustration on the part of physician and staff. When personnel policies are committed to print, they can be a major contribution to a friction-free environment in which staff members can concentrate on keeping the patient satisfied and being highly productive.

Why Bother to Print Personnel Policies?

Personnel policies set clear and high standards for the operation of your practice, as well as for staff performance, in an ever-competitive business, without forcing the doctor to be the "heavy" in day-to-day personnel issues. If one of your staff members would like a half-day off to see his or her child in a play at school, it is much easier for this issue to be dealt with through personnel policies, rather than having to say no all the time.

These policies save you valuable time because they help your office run more smoothly. With policy statements in print, you will spend less time making rulings on individual problems. When a problem arises, the staff member concerned should consult the practice's personnel statement before asking you for a ruling. Written policies serve as a "trouble shooter" to potential problems. If new personnel problems arise, they probably will not be hastily decided, because they will have to be committed to paper before being resolved.

Because personnel policies are committed to paper, careful consideration will always be given to what they say. This consideration leads to a higher standard of decisions about personnel issues. In addition, delicate issues can be better addressed and phrased in a written policy statement, and are then much less subject to interpretation.

Finally, written policies protect you against violations of the law. As you know, the labor code is becoming much more complex. For that reason, you should make sure that your policies are in compliance with the local laws pertaining to wages and work hours. You will be able to rest easier knowing that you are operating legally in the personnel area.

Components of Practice Personnel Policies

The Introduction

It is worthwhile to write an introduction to your personnel policies that illustrates how the policies relate to a concern for the needs of the patients. Explain to your staff how important these rules and regulations are and how they make it more likely that your patients will be satisfied.

General Rules

The general rules to be covered would be working hours (when you start, when you end, breaks, lunches), overtime, time record keeping, parking, vacations, holidays, sick leave, funeral leave, emergency leave,

leave of absence, personal appointments, tardiness, jury duty, and voting.

Some Policies

Determine your policies relating to pay days, termination resulting from resignation, and severance pay. A further section should cover your approach to setting wages, which generally relates to probationary periods, performance appraisals, salary increases, fringe benefits, use of office facilities and property, and so forth.

Delicate Issues

Sensitive issues that should be addressed include staff attitudes, confidentiality, patient relations, grooming, office cleanliness, smoking, personal calls, and personal activities.

Miscellaneous Issues

Such matters as accidents occurring on the premises and how travel expenses are dealt with should be covered in a section entitled miscellaneous issues.

How to Get the Project Underway

While, ideally, each policy should have the unanimous support of all the staff, it is wise to allow one person to coordinate the project, to ensure continuity and coherence throughout the manual. The coordinator could be a member of the clerical or nursing staff, or a physician. The important consideration is to ensure continuity and coherence throughout the manual.

The staff as a whole should be involved. Although the physicians will make the final decisions on policies, it can be expedient to promote staff input, since it will make later acceptance and implementation easier. Your staff will be able to highlight those areas that need discussion and consideration, and what specifically needs to be laid out.

The production of a quality finished manual involves the following ten steps:

1. Review all your current policies—both written and unwritten. This might include correspondence, memos, and oral precedents that you have set with your staff.

2. Get copies of personnel policies from other practices, companies, or a local hospital and apply these to your own situation. Make sure that these policies are in compliance with state and federal regulations.

3. Develop an overall outline of what you plan to cover in your policies. Be sure to formulate policies which are reasonable and enforceable.

4. Have the outline approved by the physicians. The key to successful implementation of policies rests with the unanimous support of the policies by all the doctors.

5. Encourage staff participation. The initial outline should be presented to staff members for their input. They should be encouraged to bring up any sensitive spots that should be addressed in the policies. Minutes should be taken of these meetings, since it may be necessary to refer to them in the future.

6. After completion, the initial outline should be written and presented to the physicians and staff for changes. It should be made clear that the physicians will make the ultimate decisions on the final product.

7. A direct writing style gets the meaning of the policies across best. Use short paragraphs with action verbs, but avoid taking a condescending tone.

8. The final product should be typed using a good-quality typewriter on 8½" × 11" paper, to be inserted in the three-ring binder that constitutes your medical office manual. Depending on the length of the final product, you may want to purchase color-coded tabs to divide the sections. Most policy statements are written in the third person; however, the pronoun *you* may be used where applicable.

9. Your staff members should each be given his or her own copies of the policy manual; each is asked to sign the master office copy.

10. Each new staff member hired should be given a copy of the policy manual and asked to sign the office copy.

Specific Considerations in Your Personnel Policy

Your Introduction

The introduction specifies the purpose of the personnel policy and explains your philosophy of the service and business aspects of medicine and your orientation toward the patient. It establishes the standards you expect your staff to achieve and states your philosophy of personnel management. A short organizational description of your practice (and possibly an organizational chart of the practice) is also included. The introduction should stress the fact that a high standard of excellence is required as it relates to the performance of each job and interactions with patients.

Conditions of Employment

The policy manual should specify if a physical examination is required of employees before they are hired to work in your office. Length of meal periods and breaks should be set, and starting/finishing times defined. The importance of punctuality and the need for staggered lunch hours should be stressed.

As a rule, most regulations require that each employee have a 15-minute break or rest period for every four hours of work. This rule varies from state to state and province to province; however, it is a handy gauge to go by.

Each job should be laid out so that a person can start and finish on time. Punctuality, of course, is critical in an office that functions well. You might consider adapting the following example to your own practice needs:

> Medical assistants are expected to be at their work stations and prepared for work, Monday through Friday, at 9 A.M., and will conclude at 6 P.M. There will be an assigned one-hour lunch period, to be taken at a time that does not interfere with patient handling. These lunch periods are not paid.
>
> A 10-minute break is permitted in the morning and a second 10-minute break in the afternoon to refresh yourself. These breaks are paid, and should be taken at your desk at a time when a break from duties will not interfere with patient flow. Lunch hours will be staggered so that someone will always be in the office to cover the telephones.
>
> It is critical that someone be there to handle the telephone during the lunch hour. Many patients cannot get away from their place of employment except during the lunch hour, and our office must be able to take these calls then. It would be a pity to miss an opportunity to bring in a new patient simply because your machine answers the telephone.

Time and Record Keeping Issues

It is law in most states and provinces that employers must keep time records. You can use either an honor system or a time clock. If you use

Figure 14-1

Time Sheet

Name of Employee _____ For Week Ending _____ 19___

Day of Week	Morning		Afternoon		Evening		Overtime		For Office Use Only		
	In	Out	In	Out	In	Out	In	Out	Regular Hours	Overtime Hours	Auth
Monday											
Tuesday											
Wednesday											
Thursday											
Friday											
Saturday											
Sunday											
Monday											
Tuesday											
Wednesday											
Thursday											
Friday											
Saturday											
Sunday											
Totals											

Overtime Report

Specific Task Breakdown		Date	Specific Work Completed	Reason for Overtime
Task	Total Time			
Subtotal				

☐ Person permitted to work overtime without special authorization

This time sheet must be personally filled out and signed by employee.

Signature _____

a sign-in time sheet, be sure it is made clear in the policy that the employee is not to round off time—for example, if someone starts at 8:55 and finishes at 5:05, those times should be recorded on the sheet, not rounded off to 9 and 5. Government auditors insist on accurate time-keeping documents. Figure 14-1 includes a sample sign-in time sheet. Note that the employees are required to sign in and out for meal periods. This allows you to curtail long lunches. Include a copy of the sign-in sheet in your policy manual in the section on record keeping.

Overtime

All overtime should be authorized in writing on your time sheet. Many times it is not easy for the employee to come to you for authorization before the fact; however, it should always be authorized on a timely basis, after the fact. It is important that all overtime be documented as to what was done and why it was necessary; this avoids the potentially uncomfortable situation in which you have to take an employee's word. Accurate, authorized overtime sheets are valuable too if you ever have to be audited.

Pay Days

The paragraph on pay days should state when pay days occur, what happens when a pay day falls on a holiday, and whether advances will be given for any reason.

Parking

The paragraph about parking should do more than assign a parking space—it should explain why the spaces close to the building are reserved for patients.

Absences

Regular attendance ensures continuity of care and service to our patients. Employees should be told that absenteeism causes disruptions and adjustments in staffing, and that employees should do whatever possible to limit absences; repeated absence without excuse is grounds for dismissal.

Sick Leave

Generally I recommend six sick days per year. After that, some practices have disability insurance that covers the employees. Sick time should be entered in the time sheet as sick leave, and be noted accordingly. Specify that sick leave may not be carried over to the following year or added to vacation time. Some practices pay for one-half of the unused sick days in order to discourage the taking of sick time. Part-timers are generally not paid sick leave.

An example of a sick leave clause might include the following:

An employee is eligible for sick leave, with pay, after three months of employment here. Six days of sick leave, with pay, are allowed per year. No more than two consecutive days are allowed without a physician's certificate. Extra time off is not granted for illness during a vacation or on a holiday. Any sick leave must be recorded on the time sheet and on the yearly calendar. Sick leave that exceeds the allotted time will be treated as time off without pay. Employees are required to call the office manager as soon as possible. Sick days may not be carried over to the next year. Payment will be made at the end of the employee's year at the rate of one-half the regular pay for days not used. Abuse of sick leave benefits could lead to dismissal.

Personal Days

There are many times when staff members need time off even though they are not sick; typically, they call in sick rather than ask for the time off, because they feel they will not get it. For this reason, I strongly urge the use of personal days; three personal days per year, which can be taken in half-day segments, would seem a reasonable amount.

Among the reasons for personal leave would be the following: emergency leave (such as the sickness of a child), funerals, voting in an election, and other miscellaneous issues.

Jury Duty

Consider developing a jury duty policy, even though the need for it arises rarely. You will be glad you have it in writing should the issue arise. Generally speaking, I recommend that you pay the difference between the employee's salary and jury pay, for up to a maximum of ten days. You should also consider how long you will hold the position open if jury duty should last for more than a specified period of time (note, however, that in many states you are required by law to keep the job open).

Vacations

In general, vacations are only given to full-time employees. They should be taken at least one week at a time, as this is truly deemed a rest. I would not recommend allowing employees to take a day here and a day there. As a rule, most offices give 10 working vacation days for one to five years of employment; 15 days for six to ten years of employment, and 20 for more than ten years.

Holidays

It is critical that you list all holidays. In some areas around the country, special state, provincial, or civic holidays are celebrated. In most instances, at least these legal holidays are observed: New Year's Day, Memorial Day, Independence Day, Labor Day, Thanksgiving, and Christmas. When one of them falls on a day when the office would ordinarily be closed (Saturday or Sunday, for example) the work day following will be considered a legal holiday for the staff, and the office will be closed.

Tardiness

It is important that employees be punctual in serving the patients' needs. Therefore, if an employee is going to be late, it is his or her responsibility to notify the immediate supervisor as soon as possible, so that someone can cover the duties. It is also important for the employees to arrive early enough to change or otherwise get ready to be at their work stations on time. Repeated tardiness (three or more time), would be potential grounds for dismissal.

Resignation

Encourage employees to give early notice of termination by paying them in full for unused sick days. Here's an example of a resignation policy:

> If you decide to resign from your position in this office, please submit written notice at least three weeks in advance of your last day at work. Compliance with this policy will make you eligible for full payment of unused sick days.

Dismissal

When writing the section on dismissal, you will find it hard to be very specific about what actions may lead to dismissal and what procedures will be followed. It should be stated that you may help an employee avoid dismissal due to incompetence by assisting her to improve her performance (that is, through performance appraisals). If a dismissal is necessary, consult Chapter 16. Dismissal may be for any of the following reasons:

1. Excessive absenteeism
2. Abuse of sick leave privileges
3. Chronic tardiness
4. Discourtesy to patients and guests at the practice
5. Inability to get along with other employees or patients
6. Willful inefficiency
7. Falsification of records
8. Dishonesty
9. Reading of patients' medical records or discussion of patients' medical conditions (except in the course of assigned duties).

Address the Types of Employment

Different types of employment in a doctor's office would include probationary, full-time, part-time, and temporary. It is critical that the personnel policies address each of these situations and discuss the rights and expectations of each. Generally speaking, part-time, probationary, and temporary employees do not enjoy any of the benefits offered by the practice.

The probationary period is usually stated as being three months from commencement of employment; employment can be terminated by either party at any time during this period.

Address the Issue of Performance Appraisals

From the outset, you should let your staff know specifically how their performance will be appraised. In order to ensure that a high quality of staff performance is maintained, it is recommended that you carefully consider Chapter 13 before you formulate your policy. One decision you need to make is whether or not the performance appraisal will affect salary increases. An example of a policy (which would be accompanied by a copy of the performance appraisal form) is the following:

The quality of your work will be evaluated twice a year by means of a performance appraisal form and interview. The purpose of this evaluation is to help you make improvements in your performance in order to maximize your potential in serving the patients of this practice.

After the goals for improvements have been agreed on, you will be given an opportunity to work toward them. Inability to make these improvements will make the employee eligible for dismissal.

Salaries

Salaries should be handled delicately, and discreetly. The following is one example of a policy regarding salaries.

Salaries are confidential and should not be discussed with other staff members. Salaries will be reviewed on the employee's anniversary date. Raises are granted according to the performance appraisal and the employee's ability to maximize patient satisfaction.

List Benefits

Many times staff do not fully realize the benefits that are paid for by the practice. These benefits should be carefully spelled out, listing each one. Some considerations would include workers' compensation that you pay on behalf of the staff member; unemployment insurance that you pay on behalf of the employee; social security that you pay on behalf of the employee; plus any other insurance, medical or dental benefits. You should specify when the employee will be eligible for various benefits, especially if such benefits accrue later on.

Key Attributes of an Effective Employee

The attributes such as personal attitudes that need to be addressed in a personnel policy manual are looked at in more depth in Chapter 13; however, they should be stressed in the personnel policies. Attitudes, as you are well aware, can have a significant effect on how well we serve our patients, as well as on fellow employees and doctors. There are many employees who do a job competently but do not project the type of attitude we want to our patients. A positive attitude, the ability to maintain confidentiality, skill in patient relations, and good personal grooming are among the important attributes an employee should have.

Attitudes

A positive attitude in dealing with patients and other staff members is critical. Since staff must often deal with irritable patients, it is essential that they maintain a pleasant, helpful attitude. Encourage staff members to respect and support each other as well as the patients, as this will provide a pleasant, reassuring atmosphere for patients. This section of a policy statement might read thus:

> Please be courteous and helpful, friendly but not familiar, as it is always a source of personal satisfaction to maintain your composure under trying and difficult conditions. Enthusiastically support the policies and reputation of this office. Reflect an attitude of cheerfulness and optimism, so that this will be a comfortable place in which to work and a satisfying and pleasant environment for our patients.

Confidentiality

A practice that radiates a feeling of trust towards its patients is likely to grow successfully. No employee can be allowed to jeopardize this trust by a breach of confidence. Stress in your policy why it is important to keep all patient information confidential. Mention, too, the consequences of not doing so. An example of a confidentiality policy might have the following:

> Information about our patients, their illnesses, and their personal lives must be kept completely confidential. When talking with a patient about any matter, try to do it in such a way that other patients in the office will not overhear. Case histories, common confidential papers, and even the appointment book should be kept where passing patients will not see them. Do not give advice to patients on personal matters, even if they ask for it. It is improper for you to reveal information concerning patients, even to another member of that patient's family, except in the case of a minor.

Patient Relations

Since your patients are your most valuable assets, emphasize to your employees that you will demand excellence in their dealings with patients. A specific policy might state:

> You are the true ambassadors of our practice. As a result, we ask that you place patient satisfaction before anything else that goes on in this

office. We are in business to please and care for our patients; anything we do should work towards that end.

Personal Grooming

In projecting a positive feeling towards patients, we must address the issue of personal grooming. When formulating this policy, you should consider having all staff members wear uniforms; if so, you must decide whether the uniforms are to be white. The policy should also state whether you will reimburse them for part of the cost, and if so, how much.

Smoking

The policy on smoking goes without saying. We are in the business of promoting good health, and we should enforce a no-smoking policy throughout the practice, except in the lunchroom during breaks. One example of a no-smoking policy is the following: "Smoking does not promote good health and is therefore not permitted in the office environment."

Personal Calls

Putting firm limits on personal calls at the start may very well save you from making unpopular decisions later. Many employees spend too much time either making or receiving personal calls when limits are not set. Permit employees to make only brief local calls and to take brief local calls that are absolutely necessary and when they do not interfere with their other duties.

Warn them to be prepared to interrupt their own call if another call comes in. An example of such a policy would include the following:

> Occasionally, personal telephone calls may have to be received or made during business hours. A small number of these will be permitted; however, they must be local calls, and must be handled so that they do not interfere in any way with your job responsibilities. Keep such calls brief, and be ready to interrupt them instantly to handle incoming calls or other office business.

Personal Activities

Since so many secondary duties to be performed in the office are put off by staff members due to lack of time, you should insist that these be done when they have a free moment. In order to maintain high standards in your office in what is rapidly becoming a competitive business, there is no time for the pursuit of personal activities by your staff. If you do not permit them to pursue personal activities at work, it is much more likely that these secondary duties will be accomplished, and in the long run your office will be a more efficient one. The policy may be as follows:

> The standards of efficiency are high in this office. There is seldom a moment when all work is completed. There is always some place in the office that needs to be reorganized or something that needs to be filed. Staff are to postpone all personal tasks until after work or until the lunch or break periods. Reading materials, such as magazines, newspapers, or books, are to be kept in the lounge and read before work or during lunchtime.
>
> Visits to the doctor and dentist should be made after hours after office hours or during lunch hours, or else a personal day from work should be taken.

Problems and Disputes

All problems and disputes should be brought to the attention of the immediate supervisor. If it cannot be resolved satisfactorily at this level, the problem should be put in writing and given to the doctors to resolve within a specific time period. Whatever ruling the doctors decide on will be carried out.

You know how important it is to have a happy, productive staff in a growing practice. To create such an atmosphere you should implement personnel policies and adhere to them. Staff members will be much happier and more productive when they understand what your policies are and what is expected of them. It is especially important that the policies tie into your practice enhancement program reason for being— which is to serve your patients.

Chapter 15

Staff Recruitment for a Competitive Edge

Patient-Oriented Staff

Your medical assistants are indeed the true ambassadors of your practice. Time invested in recruitment and interviews will pay dividends in satisfied patients and practice productivity and growth. These staff members are both the first and the last people your patients see and relate to during the visit to your office. Your patients' first contact with your practice is over the telephone with a staff member. How the call is handled, how the patient is received, and whether the patient responds to your practice with warmth are all significantly affected by how well the staff members treat your patients. Because the projection of that feeling is the very essence of the practice enhancement program, it is critical that you hire patient-centered staff members oriented toward customer service; this orientation of staff members will help you be successful in building and maintaining your practice.

Who Is That Perfect Aide?

As I guide you through the process of hiring the ideal aide, please follow sample forms (see Figures 15-1 to 15-6), which will assist you in the hiring process. Before you can hire the ideal aide, you need to decide as specifically as possible how that person walks, talks, and thinks. Figure 15-1 shows a prescreening form that helps you establish your criteria. Of course experience, education, attitude, and specific skills are critical for every job.

Practices that survive in the consumer environment are those in which staff members are oriented to customer service and project to your patients an aura of caring through their enthusiasm, warmth, and tenderness. They possess positive, healthy attitudes, and are joys to work with.

In addition to excellent social skills, of course, staff members should also be able to do the work. When necessary, they should be able to type flawlessly and quickly, handle the telephone with artistry, have impeccable handwriting, and possess good mathematical skills for insurance handling and bookkeeping. On the clinical side, they should be well trained in history taking, minor procedures, and assisting physicians.

Minimum Qualifications

As indicated, skills, attitude, and education are key in the ideal assistant. Specialized skills—such as typing, dictation, bookkeeping—and the level of competence which you expect in each area should be clearly decided, at least in your mind, from the outset. The depth of these skills depends on the amount of time that you are prepared to spend to train your new assistants, as well as on the amount of knowledge you have about current business procedures. It would be disastrous, for instance, for a physician going into his first practice, with little or no office experience, to hire an inexperienced and untrained aide. On the other hand, an experienced physician who is willing to devote some time to supervising a new assistant could make a substantial saving in the first several years by hiring an inexperienced person with excellent personal qualities.

It can be a false economy, however, to look only at the savings of a low-paid worker. One family practitioner made such a mistake as he was just beginning his practice. In the early months he was trying to

Figure **15-1**

Pre-screening Standards Form

(1) Appearance: neat & presentable

Other _____

_____

(2) Experience level

Specify _____

_____

(3) Education

Specify _____

_____

(4) Attitude: displays positive and helpful attitude

Specify _____

Other _____

_____

(5) Typing

WPM _____

Mistakes _____

(6) Dictaphone

WPM _____

Mistakes _____

(7) Application form appearance

_____

_____

(8) Other Skills

Specify _____

_____

_____

keep his cash flow as low as possible and hired a medical assistant fresh from a high school secretarial course. He felt that the savings in salary was more important than experience and skills. He had made an excellent choice in location in a high-growth area of the suburban town, and after three years his patient roster was approaching 3,000. At that point he brought me in to look at his practice, and I found that he had lost more than $15,000 because the assistant had a poor understanding of the fee schedule and could not bill the insurance companies accurately. Physicians starting in practice should hire the best; they are well worth it.

You should analyze both the needs of your practice and your own level of practice management skills in order to determine the actual qualifications of your ideal assistant. Be sure to do this before you proceed further. In hiring the aide best suited to your practice, consult the demographic study done on your area and practice. You may prefer someone who speaks more languages or fits well with the average demographic base. If you see many geriatric patients, for example, a more mature assistant might enhance your practice. In addition, you should consider the compatibility of your candidates with your present assistants if you are expanding your staff.

These steps should give you a good sense for the type of individual you are looking for, and you will have the prescreening standard form filled out.

Formulate Job Descriptions and Performance Appraisals First

After you have given ample consideration to your specific needs, it is essential that you do a job analysis in order to compose a job description for the vacant position. You know that you need a special patient-centered person in order to make your practice as successful as possible. The creation and use of a job description will be a great help in hiring the person who most closely resembles your ideal aide. Written job descriptions will also remind you what needs to be done when you are formulating your advertisement and when you are under the pressure of the interview situation.

It is also helpful for you to have your performance appraisals in place at hiring time. By preparing one in advance, you will be better able objectively to define the level of performance that you expect from your candidates. In order to gain that competitive edge, you need to consider and demand high levels of performance in specific areas. Later, during your interviews, your applicants have the right to know the level of your expectation of them.

If you take the time now to do your analysis and prepare your job descriptions and performance appraisals, you will save yourself the endless time, frustration, and expense of finding a replacement for an unsatisfactory employee.

Consult a Wide Range of Sources

In all likelihood, finding your ideal aide will require an extensive search, although it could turn out that a referral from a friend may yield the perfect employee. As many sources as possible should be consulted. It is likely that you will find her through the newspaper or from a colleague or friend, but the more creative you can get in the process, the better your long-term success.

Figure 15-2 is a recruitment sources master list, which should be assembled if possible before you need it so that it will be easy to find when the need arises. You will note that I include the telephone number, contact, and mailing address of each source. When the time comes to recruit, all you have to do is send off a letter to each particular source, or have someone call them personally. I usually suggest that your spouse or someone on your staff contact all the people on the recruitment sources list, giving them the information from your prescreening standards form, which should already have been put together.

Newspaper classified advertisements work out very well, but it is necessary to spend the extra money for an attractive presentation. I normally recommend that you use a header that is larger type, as well as a border around the advertisement, if at all possible. If you are looking for a highly skilled medical assistant, with a great deal of experience, training, and education, you should give your phone number.

You might establish a positive relationship with some medical secretarial schools by donating an hour of your time a year talking to the graduating class. This is a good way to establish rapport with the teachers and also to recruit if necessary. Another source of leads can be found in local medical secretaries associations, which are frequented by medical assistants who have an interest in their profession. Volunteering to speak at their meetings may help you find the ideal employee. Community college placement advisors can also be helpful if you have a good relationship with them; try to take the time to see them personally.

You will note that the ideal situation is to have personal contacts with people, who can lead you to a much higher caliber of personnel.

Figure **15-2**

Recruitment Sources Master List	Telephone (extension)	Contact	Mail Address
1. Newspapers			
A. _____			
B. _____			
C. _____			
D. _____			
2. Medical Secretarial Schools			
A. _____			
B. _____			
C. _____			
D. _____			
3. Local Medical Secretaries Assoc.			
A. _____			
4. Community College Placement Offices			
A. _____			
B. _____			
C. _____			
D. _____			
5. Other Secretarial Schools			
A. _____			
B. _____			
C. _____			
D. _____			
6. High Schools			
A. _____			
B. _____			
C. _____			
D. _____			
7. Colleagues			
A. _____			
B. _____			
C. _____			
D. _____			
8. Advisors (lawyers, accountants, cancellations)			
A. _____			
B. _____			
C. _____			
D. _____			

9. Hospital Personnel Departments				
A. _____				
B. _____				
C. _____				
D. _____				
10. Salespersons (Detail People and Medical Supply, other)				
A. _____				
B. _____				
C. _____				
D. _____				
11. Personnel Agencies				
A. _____				
B. _____				
C. _____				
D. _____				
12. Other Sources				
A. _____				
B. _____				
C. _____				
D. _____				

For example, detail people and medical supply salespersons have many contacts throughout many offices; they might know of a retiring physician with an excellent medical assistant who would be available for a new job.

Personnel agencies charge anywhere from 10% to 20% of the employee's first-year salary for a placement. They normally offer a guarantee for any individual they recommend. The fee can be worthwhile if you do not have the time to recruit and screen applicants properly yourself.

Compiling a master list such as this one is a one-time job that is well worth the effort, because you can use this list over and over again. If a staff vacancy occurs in the future, you can then delegate the job of notifying the sources on the master list.

You should make sure that your sources are aware of your criteria in evaluating the person who is best suited for your needs. Later, your aide can use this form to help notify the sources that you have found someone for the position when you have done so.

Prescreen Your Candidates

You need to have applications from a number of candidates to find the ideal one. Figure 15-3 is a candidate prescreening form, which is laid out so that your medical assistant or someone else can do the prescreening, to ensure that all of the initial criteria set in the job search are met before you go into the interview. This process saves your time and eliminates some of the most unlikely candidates. The prime objective in the hiring process is to screen a maximum number of candidates and devote your time to only those who have an excellent chance of being hired. My studies and past experience indicate that in an ideal practice you need to screen at least 40 candidates to find six that meet the minimum requirements for interviews. This, of course, assumes that you are looking for an exceptional medical assistant.

To facilitate the process, delegate as much as possible to others. In order to be interviewed by you, the candidate must meet the minimum qualifications you have established ahead of time. Note that the subjective evaluation of the three areas—appearance, attitude, and application form neatness—are left to the discretion of the person doing the screening. While this arrangement has often worked well and eliminated many undesirable candidates early in the process, you may want to reserve the right to make these judgments yourself. If so, you can eliminate those calls from the prescreening form.

If you have more than one assistant, you would be wise to get response from all of your staff members regarding any potential applicant, since the compatibility of your staff is an important consideration in achieving a harmonious working environment.

Setting up a typing test is a simple matter. For an applicant to type 60 words per minute (w.p.m.), in a 10-minute typing test, she must type 60×10, which equals 600 five-character words, with no mistakes. Each word can be any combinations of letters, spaces, or punctuation. (For example, the previous sentence has 67 characters, or 13.4 words.) For every mistake made, five words should be subtracted from the total number of words typed before calculating the candidate's w.p.m. score. The copy given to the candidate for the test must be typewritten.

The test should be constructed before you begin the prescreening process. The same standards can be used for dictation or shorthand. The minimum typing speed is 60 w.p.m., but a top-flight secretary can type over 100 w.p.m.

Job application forms, which are available at your local stationery stores, are fairly standard; you can modify them to meet your needs. The newer forms have a new nondiscriminatory emphasis that has no

Figure 15-3

Candidate Prescreening Form
Check (✔) if meets minimum requirements

Name	Appearance	Experience level	Education	Attitude	Typing (WPM)	Dictation (WPM)	Application form appearance	Other skills

direct references to age, marital status, race, color, or creed. The important thing to remember is that the application form should cover the main areas outlined in your prescreening form.

All candidates should be asked to handwrite their application form. Since many things in your office are handwritten, it is important that the applicant be able to write legibly. Examine the completed application form for mistakes and grammatical errors; the quality of completion of this form is a good indication of the candidate's future work. As a general rule, I never recommend doing final interviews until you have found at least three candidates who have met your minimum criteria for the office.

Telephone Interview

Figure 15-4 is an example of a telephone personality screening form. Since your medical assistants spend a lot of time talking with patients over the telephone, it is critical to know how a potential aide thinks and reacts over the telephone. It would be good to have a five-minute telephone session with all your final candidates.

Figure **15-4**

Telephone Personality Screening Form

Applicant's name _____

Rate:

	4—Excellent	2—Average	0—Poor
	3—Above Average	1—Below average	

1.	Clarity	_____
2.	Pitch	_____
3.	Speed	_____
4.	Accent	_____
5.	Pronunciation	_____
6.	Choice of words	_____
7.	Grammar	_____
8.	Sentence structure	_____
9.	Overall pleasantness	_____
	Total	_____

*Note: Must score 30–40 to qualify

When you have found the six candidates fitting the minimum criteria, your input into the interview process can begin. In addition to looking for voice clarity, pitch, speed, accent, pronunciation, choice of words, grammar, sentence structure, and overall pleasantness, you might consider how fast she thinks over the telephone. These are all good attributes to evaluate before you hire an individual. To qualify for consideration, a potential assistant should have a grade point average of 3 or above (or 30–40 points) on the telephone personality screening form.

Proper Preparation Yields Results

When you have spoken with the candidates on the telephone, done an initial evaluation, and set up a personal meeting, you are ready to begin the interviewing process. If you are equipped with your written job descriptions, performance appraisals, personnel policies, and interview questions, an in-depth interview will usually take a maximum of 45 minutes. This is time well spent when you consider the impact of this person on your patients and your practice.

Keep the objectives of the interview clear in your mind. You need to derive as much accurate information as possible about the candidates' attitudes and skills. You will also need to spend some time informing the applicant of the precise duties involved. It is necessary, but sometimes difficult, to make an accurate assessment of an applicant's experience, training, skills, and attitudes. Therefore, your questions must be designed to penetrate the candidate's "facade" and arrive at as true an evaluation as possible.

Through the use of nondirective or open-ended questions, you will usually get answers that go beyond just what the candidate feels you want to hear. You will be listening and looking for organization of thought, in addition to depth of awareness and perception. Note down what surfaces regarding personal weaknesses, as well as areas for consideration for future improvement, should you decide to hire this candidate. Specifically, you will initially be interested in understanding and knowing how the applicants perceive themselves. Some questions you might ask include:

1. What are you really good at?
2. In what areas do you feel you could improve?
3. What are your personal weaknesses?

The use of a nondirective questioning technique is also helpful in delving more deeply into the experience and education of the candidate.

In this section of the interview you will be evaluating (1) educational level; (2) experience in the medical environment; (3) self education, and (4) other relevant experience. When listening to the candidate's answers on education and experience, you should try to determine their actual quality; one way to do this is to find out how much effort it took to attain their particular level of education.

Some questions that will aid you in this evaluation are:

1. Tell me a little about your educational background and experience.
2. Are you taking any outside courses or reading anything to keep up with the current trends in physicians' offices?
3. What other experiences have you had that would help you to be a better medical assistant?

When you feel you have a good understanding of the candidate's experience and education, you are ready to proceed with a very difficult yet important aspect of the interview—an assessment of personality and attitudes. In proceeding with this part of the interview, keep in mind the personal qualities of your ideal aide. Is she positive and friendly? Does she understand that she is in a customer service business?

In measuring the candidate's personal qualities, it is especially important to assess her employment stability. It has been estimated that the cost of hiring and training a medical assistant is between one and two thousand dollars. This figure includes not only the specific cost of placing advertisements and time spent in recruiting but also the time spent in training, the cost of mistakes and "downtime" before someone leaves, and costs that relate to the hiring process. If an applicant cannot agree to a minimum of a two-year commitment to working in your office after a probationary period, you should not hire her. Some questions that will help you obtain this information are:

1. Why are you seeking a new job?
2. Why did you leave your previous job?
3. For what reasons would you consider taking a new job?

Since your aide usually creates that all-important first impression, it is essential that she be adept in handling interpersonal relations. In order to discern this ability, you might ask:

1. It's 10 o'clock. The doctor is not in yet for the 9 o'clock appointment. Three patients are waiting to see the doctor. What would you do?
2. A mother with a five-year-old child comes into the reception area. The child is obviously upset about seeing the doctor. What would you do?

3. What do you think the role of the medical assistant is in relationship to the patient?

Because your aide will probably have a variety of duties to perform,
often under the pressure of an ever-ringing telephone or a crowded
reception room, it is important that she have enough organizational
ability to both understand and carry out her priorities. To get a feeling
for this organizational ability, you might inquire:

1. How would you go about setting up my office if I were just beginning my practice?
2. What advice would you give me?
3. Can you relate a personal experience to me where you organized
something that you're really proud of?

During times of great stress or emergency in the office, an intelligent
aide may prove invaluable. Although you will have a feeling for the
candidate's intelligence already, you will get a more accurate picture by
asking her what she would do if a patient came into the office bleeding
and in great pain and she was the only one there. You probably already
have her academic record; ask her about any low grades she received.

In conjunction with intelligence and experience, alertness is an
important quality in keeping your office progressive and productive. You
might ask her what she saw in the office that could be improved, and
what in the office she really liked or disliked.

While initiative in completing tasks are important, conscientiousness
and thoroughness in carrying them out are essential in the medical
assistant's position. To assess her ability to handle detail and complete
tasks accurately, you might ask her to evaluate herself on a scale of 1
to 10 for being conscientious and thorough. Ask her to give examples
that demonstrate these traits.

Most personnel experts say that maturity is a desirable attribute of
a productive, well-adjusted employee. You might ask:

1. How would you define a mature person?
2. Within your definition, how would you rate yourself?
3. How would you handle a belligerent caller who is badgering you
about what he claims is an incorrect balance on his bill, when
your calculations show that the bill is correct, but he is not prepared to listen to you?

Staff members with a positive approach to life can interact
successfully with your patients and with you. These positive attitudes
allow them to see problems as "improvable situations," and view

Figure **15-5**

Personal Interview Evaluation Form

Applicant's Name _____

Rate: 4—Excellent   1—Below average
                         3—Above average   0—Poor
                         2—Average

A. General appearance
    (a) poise   _____
    (b) grooming   _____
    (c) dress   _____
    (d) mannerisms   _____
B. Voice
    (a) diction   _____
    (b) articulation   _____
    (c) fluency of speech   _____
    (d) proper grammer   _____
C. Job skills
    (a) typing   _____
    (b) dictation   _____
    (c) legibility of handwriting   _____
    (d) other skills   _____
D. Experience and education
    (a) education level   _____
    (b) experience in medical environment   _____
    (c) self education   _____
    (d) other relevant experiences   _____
E. Attitudes and personal attributes
    (a) employment stability   _____
    (b) interpersonal relations   _____
    (c) organization ability   _____
    (d) intelligence   _____
    (e) conscientiousness & thoroughness   _____
    (f) initiative & leadership   _____
    (g) maturity   _____
    (h) positive attitude (enthusiasm)   _____
    (i) alertness   _____
    (j) orientation to patients   _____

    Total   _____

Note: Must score 80–100 to qualify

---

obstacles as mere challenges to overcome. Positive people gravitate toward success, and they are a joy to work with. Some questions to determine whether or not a candidate has such attitudes include the following:

1. What did you like about your last job?
2. What did you dislike about your last job?
3. It's 7 P.M. on a Friday. You have had the worst day in the office in six months. Patients are crowding the examination room, and you have an important event to attend. What would you do?

As you can see, an employment interview must cover a number of issues—with patient orientation and caring being the most important. However, this is not the only aspect of the interview. You also need to give a specific description of your expectations to the potential candidate for the job. The more information you can give the potential job candidate during the interview, the better. Discuss in detail the job descriptions, performance appraisals, and personnel policies. Keep in mind that you are beginning a potential relationship that may last for many years so try to start out on the right foot. Make sure you ask candidates whether they have any questions or comments, and let them know when you will be getting back to them regarding their status as potential employees.

Try to do as little writing as possible during the interview, because this is disruptive to the candidate as well as to yourself. When you have completed the interview, take a few minutes to fill in all the ratings on the personal interview evaluation form (see figure 15-5).

Discuss Salary Benefits and Duties

Besides being an evaluation process, the interview is also a fact-finding process for the employee, who will ask questions regarding duties, salary, and personnel policies. These should be answered frankly; however, you should schedule a final meeting before you hire someone permanently, to carefully go over each salary and personnel policy issue.

Check Those References

After you have interviewed all candidates, choose the top two or three in terms of scores from the interview evaluation form for the telephone reference checking. This is a vital step in the hiring process; it takes only 10 minutes per applicant yet yields great value. There is a

Figure 15-6

Telephone Reference Checking Questionnaire

Applicant's Name _____ Telephone _____ Check

Person Contacted _____ Question

Position _____

1. Skills—How did you find the quality and speed of work in the following areas:
   (1) Typing? _____
   (2) Dictation? _____
   (3) Other? _____

2. Personality and attitudes
   (a) Employment stability
       —How long did she work with you? _____
       —Why did she leave? _____
   (b) Interest in people
       —Did she interelate well with:
       (1) your patients? _____
       (2) your staff? _____
   (c) Organizational ability —Was she well organized? _____
   (d) Intelligence —Did she come up with useful suggestions to improve the office? _____
       —Could she solve prolems without a lot of interaction with you? _____
   (e) Conscientiousness and thoroughness —Was she conscientious? _____
       —Did she complete her work thoroughly? _____
   (f) Initiative and leadership —Did she create useful projects for herself and complete them? _____
       —Would you say she has good leadership capabilities? _____
       —As situations arose did she handle them with maturity and good judgment? _____
   (g) Maturity
   (h) Positive attitude —Was she cheerful and enthusiastic about her work and the people around her? _____
   (i) Alertness —Was she usually attentive and alert? _____

3. Evaluation
   (a) Was she punctual? _____
   (b) Did she have good attendance? _____
   (c) What was her main faults? _____
   (d) What was the most significant problem you have had with the person? _____
   (e) Would you rehire her? _____

great difference between meeting someone for a 45-minute interview and knowing or working with this person over a long period of time. Who knows the on-the-job capabilities and attitudes of an applicant better than a former employer? The telephone reference checking questionnaire in Figure 15-6, which is designed to corroborate the interview evaluation form, will help you see how well your opinion of the candidate is supported by past employers.

It is wise to call at least two reference sources, preferably ones that are work related. When you have completed the reference checks, you should be ready to make your final decision.

The Moment of Truth

You are now ready to make your final choice. You know that your ideal ambassador is bright, friendly, tactful, enthusiastic, positive, professional, and competent. She will contribute a positive and professional air to your practice. Yes, she has a few weaknesses; however, you know what they are and have a pretty good idea that she will improve and that you can help her eventually overcome them. She is exceptional at greeting your patients because she knows how important it is that she please your customers. She will deal with her office duties competently and enthusiastically and will ask for payment confidently and tactfully.

Never make the final choice on the spot; at least give it one night's sleep if possible, and discuss it with as many people as you can before you make the final decision. Have the rest of your staff, or your adviser, interview your candidate if possible. When you reach consensus after thoroughly going through the process, you should have found an ideal candidate to assist you in implementing and updating your practice enhancement program.

Chapter 16

Terminating Staff Members

There will almost certainly come a time when you have to dismiss an unsatisfactory employee. The process is never pleasant, but your approach to it can make an important difference in the long-term success of your practice. The following cautionary story shows how *not* to go about firing an employee.

It was a crisp, icy morning in the new year. With resolution, Dr. Coldstone donned his black suit and power tie. Arriving at his office at 8.55 A.M., he promptly summoned Mary Smith, his receptionist of two years. As her voice pierced the silence of the sterile business area with a brisk "Good morning," the words froze in her throat, for before her, on his desk, was her employee file folder.

Immediately she knew that the inevitable was about to happen. She had been aware from the grunts and the cold shoulder the doctor had been giving her during the past few months that he had been irritated by her difficulties in dealing with the additional influx of patients generated by his new referral sources. Still, he was being unreasonable, she felt. After all, was it her fault that some telephone calls were being lost because she had to cope with a waiting room full of restless, whining children. Was it her fault that she often didn't have time to ask patients for payment at the time of service—when they didn't want to pay anyway? And was it her fault that she didn't have time to clear off her desk and get organized?

137

As hard as it was for her to believe, this was really it. His words, "I have to fire you, Mary. I just can't cope with your incompetence any longer. Consider this your two weeks' notice, and I would appreciate your cooperation with the new girl," echoed through her mind all morning. How could he do such a thing without trying to help her first? Who did he think he was? No one could get away with treating Mary Smith like that. She'd fix him!

Six weeks later, when the efficient new medical secretary began to settle in, she discovered that a number of items were missing. Most notable were several accounts receivable cards and charts. This presented problems, since there was no way to determine all the patients who had been removed from the system. Many months later, Dr. Coldstone and his accountant realized that this act of negligence, which could be pinned on no one, had cost him as much as $15,000.

Although Dr. Coldstone was atypical in his lack of sensitivity in firing his receptionist, he was like many busy physicians who do not understand that the termination of an employee must be done carefully. When performed artfully, this process can rid you of unsatisfactory employees without incurring their wrath and subsequent revenge.

Basic Considerations in Deciding Whom to Terminate and Why

If you run your practice on the premise that the main purpose of staff members is to create and maintain a high level of patient satisfaction, then anyone who persistently fails to live up to the role of practice ambassador ought to be replaced by someone who can and will. Employees may fail to be excellent ambassadors in the following circumstances:

1. They persistently do not obey the rules and regulations, as laid out in your personnel policy manual for their benefit and the benefit of the patients.
2. They do not perform some aspect of their job, as detailed in their job description, to a high level to serve the patient.
3. They do not meet your performance or attitudinal standards, as described in your performance appraisal.

In these times of physician competition, cost control and changing patient attitudes you cannot afford to employ an assistant who is not committed to meeting the needs of your patients.

Although the actual act of termination is never a pleasant one, the unpleasantness is soon forgotten when you replace your substandard employee with a pleasing and productive one.

The Borderline Ambassador

Only occasionally does an employee break a rule, such as a breach of confidentiality, that requires an immediate dismissal. By far the most common and complex problem is that of the employee who meets your standards part of the time. One physician, for example, had an assistant who was in many ways an ideal hostess and ambassador to the patients. She was always pleasant when patients arrived, and smiled and reassured them whenever she could. However, she could never get the new scheduling system right. As a result, patients were often incorrectly booked, and her employer was often left twiddling his thumbs and waiting for a new patient to come in. A new appointment scheduling system had been implemented. The doctor worked with the assistant on a number of occasions, and when he was supervising her closely she got it right. Left on her own devices, however, she always got it wrong.

It is difficult when an employee who performs adequately on one part of the job causes a number of additional problems in another of her functions. In this case you would make your judgment on whether you feel the employee might be able to improve her all-round performance to meet the standard demanded.

Firing the Long-term Employee

Many times long-term employees can develop problems over the years—for example, they may become alcoholics, develop poor attitudes (possibly as a result of personal crises), or be distracted by a change in marital status or family situation. Sometimes these situations can be improved through a dedicated effort by both parties, and sometimes through the evaluation process you will realize that a termination interview must be conducted.

The Point of Firing

With every employee, you have basically two clear-cut alternatives (a third alternative is available, but I do not recommend it). Alternative

1 is to fire any employee who is not working to the standard you feel is necessary to keep your patients satisfied. Alternative 2 is that both you and the employee work aggressively to improve his or her performance to meet the desired level. Alternative 3 is to do nothing.

Most physicians choose number 3. A number of employees do not meet the standards that would provide a high level of service to patients and yet we continue to subsidize their ineptitude far beyond a reasonable time for improvement.

Keeping Your Options Open

It is critical that you follow a well-planned termination process, which is important for two reasons: (1) it allows you to make a break without any major office repercussions, and (2) it keeps you covered legally. Lawsuits can be expensive and time consuming; in addition you do not want to have the unpleasantness of a complaint filed against you with the fair labor and standards group in your area.

Steps in the Dismissal

Step 1—Probationary period. You need to ensure that you have a probationary period for every employee you hire. I recommend that each new person be asked to work for a prehiring period of several days as part of the interview process, before you even consider hiring them.

Once you have decided to hire the person, she should be put on a three-month probationary period. If the performance is not satisfactory within that period, dismissal is much easier while the assistant is still a stranger than after you have gotten to know her. If the person is marginal, it is better to drop her now or else extend the probationary period. Do not, however, extend anyone's probationary period more than once.

Step 2—Regular performance appraisals. Regular performance appraisals with all employees are important because they help you focus on those areas that need improvement. The appraisal sessions provide you and your employee an opportunity to discuss your expectations and her ability to fulfill those expectations. If the employee gives you a plausible excuse for poor performance, set down in writing plans for bringing about improvement, and mark a date on your calendar to review the situation. Normally, employees should be willing to improve their performance within an agreed-upon time frame.

Make sure you document all the performance appraisals. This is critical in the evaluation process.

Step 3—Withholding salary increases. Until performance improves, you should not increase the assistant's salary because a salary increase should be related to satisfactory performance. Many times, the employee may decide to quit because a salary increase was withheld—this will save you the aggravation of the termination procedure later.

Step 4—Accept any resignation. If an employee ever offers to resign, always accept the resignation; anyone who wants to quit is not committed to meeting your standards. Give her vacation and severance pay, and relieve her of her duties as soon as you can find a replacement.

*Step 5—Begin the hiring process.*Make sure you are equipped to deal with the departure of an unsatisfactory employee. As soon as you notice that she is not meeting the standards that your agreed on (as reviewed during different approaches), you should begin the hiring interview process.

When advertising for applicants, use a box number and have the applications sent to your house. Conduct the interviews at some place other than the office, and be prepared to bring a new person in as soon as you have made your decision. You should never be left without coverage in your office; otherwise, you are likely to make a bad decision while under the pressure of having to act quickly.

Step 6—Prepare for effect on staff morale. If you have a supervisor in the office, inform that person that it is not necessary to tell other staff members the reason for the employee's termination. Let her know that she will be temporarily assuming some extra responsibilities. Try to keep the termination process from spoiling any positive morale that you have built up in the office. No matter how much an assistant may be disliked, she will be missed when terminated.

*Step 7—Share the decision.*Reach a unanimous decision with any partners you may have prior to making a decision to terminate an employee. This will lessen the chance that your assistant will consult any of them seeking support. By ensuring that you have the full agreement of your partners in this decision you know you will have their backing if problems arise later.

Step 8—Amount of notice. Decide whether to give two weeks' notice, or whether the employee should leave immediately after the interview. Generally it seems preferable to release the terminated employee immediately, giving her the two weeks severance pay; this avoids the possibility that an employee might try to damage your practice after the decision to terminate her has been made. (if Dr. Coldstone had done this, the assistant would not have had time to plan repercussions to the practice). There is always a danger, too, that a terminated employee might stir negative morale in the office before leaving.

Step 9—Follow written procedures. You should strictly adhere to the termination process detailed in your manual to avoid legal action.

Step 10—Documentation. Always keep the discharged employee's personnel records, and even more important, the performance appraisals, in case a legal problem should arise in the future.

Prepare for the Termination Interview

A well-laid out interview will go smoothly. Like any well-run meeting, it should have an agenda. If you have a clear plan, you will be able to deal better with the fact that your decision to terminate is definite and final.

There are some details you should remember in the termination process: (1) The check should be made out to cover the salary due, as well as unused vacation pay and termination pay (unless your manual specifies otherwise, the termination pay is for two weeks). (2) Prepare a letter of reference. Even if you can find nothing for which to praise the employee, you can at least confirm that she was employed by you for a specific period of time. If you decide to elaborate on her work in a letter, be honest; do not write anything you do not believe. Have the check, the letter, and her personnel file at hand at the final interview.

How to Conduct the Interview

Conduct the termination in a professional manner. Be calm and courteous, no matter what. In an honest but kind manner, you should follow these steps:

1. Plan to be firm in order to let the employee know that the termination is final. Begin by reminding her that you had set this time six months previously to review her performance. Tell her you had made it clear that if you were not satisfied by now you would terminate the employment. State emphatically that you are not satisfied, and therefore you are terminating her. Tell her you have her check, and explain how you arrived at that amount. Tell her also that she can use the free time allotted by the severance

pay to find a new job, and that it will be more comfortable for her that way, rather than to continue in her present role.

2. Let the employee respond. While she is doing so, keep in mind that being fired is a crushing experience. Enumerate her good points, but do not hesitate to tell her the truth—she needs to know it. Anyone whose performance justifies a dismissal is entitled to know the real reason. You might make a suggestion about a line of work in which she might do well.

3. Try to conclude the interview on a positive note, and offer her your best wishes.

Your staff members, as has been emphasized earlier, are the ambassadors of your practice. They are responsible for all the details that keep the patient satisfied. You should never lower your standards and put up with an employee who is not a worthy representative of your practice. A key principle of practice enhancement is that your patients deserve nothing but the best.

Your Practice

To succeed in a competitive era physicians will be reassessing, refining, changing, and implementing more efficient office systems and procedures. The well-organized and smooth-running medical office will help make patients feel that physicians and staff are a competent and caring team; this will inspire their trust, cooperation, and patronage. Improvement in office systems and procedures will also be more professionally satisfying and rewarding for you.

The delicate balance between efficiency and patient service will be examined in this section. Your systems should be structured so you can work close to your most efficient level 100 percent of the time. This can only be achieved by careful delegation to well-trained staff members and through use of quality systems. Chapter 17 discusses the trade-off between efficiency and patient service.

Essential to the maximization of your time and productivity is the implementation of an effective appointment scheduling system tailored to the specific needs of your practice. Inefficient appointment scheduling, more than any other practice variable, causes the majority of patient complaints. Chapters 18–20 present a fresh approach to developing a customized schedule and offer techniques to minimize problems in this area.

Patient compliance and orientation are critical to a smooth-functioning practice. Your printed informational materials, particularly a patient information booklet, can do much to help you project your practice to your patients with tact and with a positive attitude. Chapter 21 shows you how to develop patient information booklets to present your practice positively.

Good public relations is very important in the service business, and of course, your telephone is the lifeline to your practice as well as the patient's first contact with the practice. Chapter 22 shows you how to manage the telephone in a way that improves your patients' perceptions of your practice.

Well-organized medical records and charting procedures are key systems that needs to be well-integrated into the practice. Patients get better care and better treatment from the staff if your records system is well thought out. Chapter 23 looks at some of the current thinking on charting and records management.

Collections and financial control is an area that needs to be readdressed in a competitive era. Systems that worked well in the past need to be readapted to contemporary pricing realities. Chapter 24 covers some key considerations in your collections systems.

Financial accounting is another area that needs your close attention. In order to make prudent decisions relating to quality and cost, you must develop an effective management system that lets you know how your practice is running. Chapter 26 describes some concepts in financial accounting that will help you stay competitive.

Finally, creating a pleasant environment in which to deliver care calls for careful planning of your facility to project an image of efficiency and caring to your patients. In a competitive era, it is important to design facilities that enable you to deliver care to your patients comfortably and effectively. Some new design concepts and current thinking about facility planning are discussed in Chapter 25.

In the past a practice could grow without good practice management systems, but it is now critical to ensure that good systems are effectively integrated within your total practice enhancement program. Your future depends on it.

━━━━━━━━━━━━━━━━━━━━━━━━━━━━━━━━━━●

Chapter 17

How to Improve Physician and Staff Productivity Without Sacrificing Patient Service

Satisfying patients requires more than simply treating their medical problems. In order to build a viable practice in these competitive times, it is critical that your office be as productive and efficient as possible, in order to provide high-quality, cost-effective care. There is a delicate balance between a satisfied patient and efficiency. You may be able, for example, to diagnose and treat a patient's problem in less than five minutes; however, if proper attention is not given to the quality of the social interaction, the patient may feel that the doctor spent too little time on his or her problem.

When surveys are made of practices, the patients are asked for feedback about the practice. One question that would routinely be asked of patients is "Do you feel that the doctor spends enough time with you?" The answers to this question can give valuable insight into the importance of the social interaction. In one city, surveys of two internal medicine practices yielded startling results. One internist spent 25 percent more time with patients, yet he consistently achieved lower scores on that

149

question. Examination of the styles of both physicians revealed that the better-ranked doctor had effective systems and procedures in place, so that she did not waste a minute. Her prescription pads were preprinted for high-frequency prescriptions, and she used dictation equipment and staff effectively. She was able to spend more time on socialization, even though she decreased the total time of the visit through the use of effective systems and procedures and delegation. Although the second doctor spent more time with patients, he lost a lot of time making handwritten notes and filling out parts of insurance forms during the visit. It was the delicate balance between efficiency and patient service that made the difference.

By making the best use of your own time, you will increase your output. The improvement of your own productivity will be professionally, personally, and financially rewarding. It will also benefit your patients: when you and your practice are more efficient and productive, you will be able to deliver a consistent, high level of service that is still cost effective.

You can only maximize your time by establishing the appropriate systems and procedures to make your staff more efficient and productive. Improving your staff's overall efficiency and productivity will also directly benefit your patients. Since your staff is part of the overhead of the practice, patient care costs will be stabilized through efficient systems and procedures that reduce the need for more staff. For example, if you have an excellent billing system in place, your bills will get out in a timely manner with less reliance on staff time.

The Delicate Balance

How can you make yourself more productive and still give high quality service? The first tenet is to manage your time so that you can work at your most efficient level. You must develop the ability to delegate wisely, implement effective practice management and procedures, and have the best possible facilities and equipment to allow you to work as efficiently as possible. When the appropriate systems and procedures are in place, you and your staff members have more time to deliver the service your patients are learning to expect.

Appreciate the Value of Your Time

Table 17-1 is a breakdown to determine what your time is worth. Based on working 48 weeks per year, five days per week, at 10 hours

Table 17-1
The value of your time.[a]

If You Gross	Each Minute Is Worth	Each Hour Is Worth	10 Minutes a Day Turned Productive Is Worth Per Year	Value of 10[b] Productive Minutes Over Ten Years
$25,000/yr.	$0.17	$10.20	$408,00	$6,502
50,000/yr.	0.35	21.00	840.00	13,387
75,000/yr.	0.52	31.20	1,248.00	19,889
100,000/yr.	0.70	42.00	1,680.00	26,774
125,000/yr.	0.87	52.20	2,080.00	33,276
150,000/yr.	1.04	63.00	2,496.00	39,778
200,000/yr.	1.40	84.00	3,360.00	53,548
250,000	1.74	104.40	4,176.00	66,553
500,000/yr.	3.48	208.80	8,352.00	133,105

[a]Based on 48 weeks, 5 days a week, 10 hours a day.
[b]Value of fund before taxes, assuming a 10% interest rate, compounded annually.

per day, if you gross $100,000 annually, each minute is worth 70 cents.

How do you reconcile, then, that when you are seeing patients or performing surgery you are earning significantly more money per patient care hour? This relates specifically to the fact that you perform a number of tasks through the day that are not at your highest level. If you have been performing a number of nonremunerative duties and lower-level tasks, such as driving between office and hospital, performing administrative duties around the office, cleaning up the examination rooms, doing preliminary histories and vital signs, and carrying out such minor procedures as injections, you will lower your average hourly pay. Neither you nor your patients will benefit from your performing at lower levels; therefore, you owe it to yourself and to your patients to watch every minute of your time.

Understanding the Levels of Work in Your Practice

To understand the practice management aspects of your practice enhancement program in your office, you will need to break down all the key tasks performed in a medical office. This will not only focus your attention on how you work, it will also enable you to understand the relative values of various tasks in the office, thus helping to establish your priorities and ensure that everyone in the office is working at their most efficient level. Generally, these categories can be divided into five levels.

Level 5 represents those tasks that require a physician, including such duties as nonroutine history taking, physical examination, analysis and diagnosis, and treatment, as well as motivating on patient education. This is what you went to medical school for, this is what you do best, and this is what is exciting about the practice of medicine. As a rule, all level 5 tasks can only be done by a physician and cannot be delegated except in very specialized situations.

Level 4 tasks are those that are important in the treatment and diagnosis of patients, but can, at your discretion, be delegated to well-trained paramedical assistants who can carry out these procedures at a much lower hourly cost. These tasks would include preliminary history taking, preliminary testing, minor treatment, routine patient education and counseling, patient follow-up, and injections. Although you can perform all these tasks during the "socialization" period with patients, they can be delegated if it fits your style of practice.

Level 3 clinical tasks, which could be performed by medical assistants with little clinical training, include: preparing and cleaning up the treatment room, initial interview for the chief complaint, taking vital signs, weigh ins, sterilizing instruments, and general cleanup. Ordinarily we categorize these by asking the question: Could an intelligent person be trained to handle any of these paramedical tasks?

Level 2 includes the secretarial and administrative tasks that requires a trained secretary. Such duties as banking, bookkeeping, payroll, ordering supplies, scheduling appointments, writing letters, handling accounts receivable, answering the telephone, and typing dictation or copy are nonclinical in nature; however, they do require a level of secretarial experience or training.

Level 1 represents those clerical tasks that can be performed by someone with little or no training, under supervision. They include such items as filling out the routine aspects of insurance forms; opening and processing mail; pulling and filing charts; filing reports, opening patient charts, miscellaneous filing, housekeeping, and straight copy typing. As you can see, these tasks can normally be performed by a low-cost clerk.

Some physicians still personally perform Level 1 to Level 4 tasks in their practices. By doing so, they are diminishing their own productivity, effectiveness, and output. They are, in fact, lowering their dollar per hour value. For example, if you gross $200,000 per year, and work 10 hours a day during a five day week, for 48 weeks of the year, your average hourly gross is $84. However, if you are carrying out surgical procedures and seeing patients, you are grossing much higher than this $84 per hour figure. The lower overall average relates directly to the fact that you are performing a number of nonremunerative and less productive tasks.

A case could be made that a number of these lower-level jobs are performed during the time of socialization with the patient. Using this thinking will allow you to rationalize doing such tasks; however, I maintain that you can do a better job of socialization if you are not distracted by other things. It is far better to concentrate on the patient and to work at a higher level in the critical interaction with and education of the patient, rather than to perform those other distracting and lower-cost duties.

Medical practitioners must begin to think of efficiency and productivity as they move into these competitive times. As price competition begins to affect the system, more attention will be placed on the effective and efficient delivery of care. Also, efficient practices exude a level of confidence to the patient, which gives such practices the competitive edge.

Maximize Your Time

The key principle to maximizing your time in your office is to ensure that you are working at your most efficient level—Level 5. Make an active effort, therefore, to delegate as much of the other levels of work as possible.

In many large corporate organizations, executives who are earning $50 an hour spend virtually 100 percent of their time doing work at that level. These companies realize that the value they receive from highly paid executives comes only when these executives are doing the level of work they are being paid to do. Therefore, such companies make sure that highly trained assistants and good secretarial support are always available, and that all the equipment needed to perform the work is at hand.

As you can see, if you make 10 extra minutes per day productive and invest the 10 minutes, at $100,000 per year you would have saved $1,680.00. Over a 10-year period, assuming a 10 percent interest rate, if 10 additional minutes were turned productive you would have a fund of $26,774, which is a sizable step toward your retirement fund or your children's education—or toward owning a Mercedes.

As you delegate more and more of the Level 1 to Level 4 tasks and you are operating more frequently at your most challenging level (Level 5), you will be devoting more time to the sharpening and refining of the medical skills you were trained for. Not only will performing at your highest level be more professionally satisfying, but you are likely to be a sharper doctor—with benefits that affect both yourself and your patient. Patients will have more quality time with you when a caring and well-trained member of your staff does some of the minor clinical procedures.

Delegate your reading. One of my clients delegates all his reading to a high-level nurse. He pays her well, but feels she is worth it, because she goes through all the journals and magazines and clips anything he might want to read. After all, more time is spent in flipping pages than in looking at the "meat" of the publication. He then reviews a scrap book of critical ideas without having to wade through piles of heavy journals. (Other delegation techniques will be discussed further in the last chapters of this text.)

Use *preprinted prescription pads.* Eighty percent of all prescriptions in your practice are written for 20 scripts. Have these preprinted, and all you need do is sign them as they are needed.

Do dictation while you are traveling. This makes good use of your travel time and increases your daily output.

Listen to tapes on medical education as you travel instead of doing it during your own personal time.

Consider prepared rubber stamps for notes in your chart. This can save a great deal of writing.

Use *dictation equipment* rather than writing notes on patient charts.

Consider using *videotape presentations* on patient education topics that you find yourself discussing over and over. Thus, your patients can be viewing you on a monitor while you see another patient.

Make sure you have *efficient systems and procedures* in place for appointment scheduling, telephone calls, writing routine letters, and so forth.

Make sure that you have *well-trained staff members* able to execute your systems, and procedures; they should be familiar with your policies.

Plan your facility with as much time savings in mind as possible.

In my experience, successful medical practitioners who utilize their time judiciously are able to provide optimum patient care and achieve maximum professional, personal, and financial satisfaction. Now is the time to do some critical thinking and chart a positive course of action toward maximizing your output and maintaining control of your professional and personal life.

━━━━━━━━━━━━━━━━━━━━━━━━━━━━━━━━━━━━━━━●

Chapter 18

Creative Scheduling Techniques

An interesting fad is emerging around the country: Patients are suing their doctors for excessive waiting time, and, amazingly, they are winning. In the last year, a number of patients took their doctors to small claims court for what they considered excessive time spent waiting for service. Although it might seem a little extreme, this fact shows how important appointment scheduling is to your patients.

You will find that seeing patients on time is a valuable asset in building your practice and will give you a competitive advantage in an area that is deficient in most medical practices. More than any other aspect of practice management, appointment scheduling is one that needs to be squarely addressed. Physicians who are consistently able to see their patients on time will reap significant benefits in patient referrals and practice growth. Scheduling problems can exact a personal cost to you because they prevent you from being home on time. They can also take a financial toll because they invariably leave you with unhappy patients, some of whom will leave your practice. Finally, seeing patients on time can also result in your being able to see more patients, which, in turn, is profitable for you.

Have you ever stopped to consider why your appointments run late? A dozen or more recurring problems can result in this situation. When you examine these problems carefully, you will find that they can be rectified.

Analyze Your Attitudes Toward Time

Practices that are regularly behind schedule are usually so because of the physician's attitude regarding time. If you view your patients' time as valuable and make a concerted effort to see them on schedule, you should be successful. My experience shows that you should be able to see 80 percent of your patients within 10 minutes of their assigned appointment time; this means, on the other hand, that you will generally see 20 percent of your patients late.

Causes of Scheduling Problems

If you see most of your patients late, then you need to do some analysis. To begin, you should examine closely the factors that relate to your being behind. Some of the most frequent problems will be discussed in the following sections.

Emergencies

In general you might say that emergencies cannot be scheduled. However, you might find that you have more emergencies on Mondays and Fridays than on other days of the week. If your practice is located in a highly industrialized area, emergencies may be more frequent during the last few hours of the afternoon. As a rule, you will be able to identify a pattern in which emergencies occur more often on particular days or at particular times. If you can determine the pattern, you should schedule fewer appointments during times when emergencies are apt to occur.

The Tardy Doctor

Medical assistants report that more than any other aspect of the time problem, the tardy doctor is the worst offender. Such tardiness is attributable both to the large demands on a doctor's time and to the doctor's attitude about seeing patients.

A number of solutions are available for keeping physicians on time, especially when they are out of the office. One physician had a standing rule that his medical assistant should page him 45 minutes before he was due in the office. In addition to acting as a reminder, this enabled the doctor to begin the sequence of going to the telephone and then to the office. Some receptionists compensate for the physician's tardiness by scheduling fewer appointments at the beginning of the day, as well as by scheduling those patients who are least likely to mind waiting at the end of the morning or afternoon.

When you are late, your patients should be told how late you are likely to be and given an opportunity to reschedule their appointments. If possible, your medical assistant should call patients in advance and advise them that you are running late. In this way you are letting your patients know that you care about them, that you realize their time is valuable, and that you regret the delay.

One way of cutting down on your time at the hospital is to visit the doctors' lounge *before* doing your rounds. Thus, you will be less likely to get caught up in discussions with other physicians.

Walk-ins and Work-ins

Walk-ins and work-ins, two of the key destroyers of your schedule, cause an uneven day and disrupt everyone's schedule for the rest of the day. A number of these patients represent actual or possible emergencies, of course, and therefore the nurse should screen all walk-ins to determine the nature of the problem. Only emergencies should be handled immediately. If the case is not an emergency, the patient should be rescheduled for a later time. This reinforces the appointment system and gently forces the patients to use it.

One young doctor who bought a practice from an elderly family practitioner had to devise a plan to introduce an appointment schedule to patients used to being able to see the doctor on a walk-in basis. The new doctor put up two large clocks similar to those used in grade schools. Under one clock is written, "Next patient walk-in will be seen at X time." Under the second clock are the words, "Next patient with appointment will be seen at Y time." Walk-ins and work-ins are handled on a predetermined basis of one walk-in per hour, and patients with appointments always get priority. The clocks usually show a three-hour difference (favoring the patients with appointments). Therefore, a walk-in can clearly see that there is an advantage to making an appointment.

A Texas internist has a daily walk-in clinic that allows patients to see him for a short one- to five-minute period between the hours of 4 and 5 P.M. every day, without calling ahead of time. This allows patients to see the doctor for minor problems—prescription renewals and other such limited needs—and improves the doctor's accessibility.

One group practice in Boston arranges its schedule so that the doctor on call has no patients from 4 to 5 P.M. and takes care of all the walk-ins during that time. Another group in Florida designates a "floating" physician who is assigned the light patient load for that day; all walk-ins and work-ins are directed to this physician.

It is wise to encourage your patients to call before dropping in. Tell them that you may be able to work them in, but they should be prepared to wait unless they have an emergency.

No-Shows

Patients who fail to show up for their appointments can destroy a schedule. Your time is valuable too. The open time that such patients create may well have been used for walk-in and emergency patients.

There are a number of specific solutions to this regular problem. If, for example, the patient in question is known to be a new patient, is coming in with a specific condition or problem (for example, diabetes), or has an appointment for an annual check-up, you can schedule the appropriate laboratory tests one week before the examination. (Do not forget to tell the patient to go to the laboratory instead of to your office.) The benefit of this arrangement is that the test results will be on hand at the time of the office visit; it also reminds patients that they have an appointment with you. If the patient misses the laboratory visit, have your assistant cancel the patient's appointment with you and reschedule the tests. For legal purposes, keep a record of all patients who fail to keep their appointments.

Reminders

You should also use the telephone reminder system. When patients call for an appointment, get telephone numbers at which they can be reached during days and evenings. The day before the appointment, have your assistant call and remind them of their visit. Also, make sure that patients are given an appointment card reminding them of their next visit. To increase the likelihood that they will save these cards, include such information as blood type, drug allergies, and immunization histories on them. Because the cards carry important medical information, the patients are less likely to throw them out or misplace them. Some practitioners mail reminder cards. When an appointment is made out for a specified date, the patients put their names and addresses on a post card. The card is then filed in a calendar file so that it is placed in the mail one week before the appointment date.

Latecomers

One specialist who had a serious problem with latecomers used several approaches to alleviate this problem. He had his assistants make telephone reminders. In addition, he used the "wave" system for scheduling surgical visits; that is, he saw six patients per hour, scheduling two patients on the hour, one patient at quarter past the hour, two more at half past the hour, and another at 15 minutes before the hour. Thus he always had a reservoir of patients in the reception room, so that if patients were late he had less to worry about. He also highlighted charts of consistent latecomers and regularly gave them the last appointment of the morning or the afternoon, when he usually was behind anyway. Ultimately, he did have to make a formal termination of the physician-patient relationship with a few chronic latecomers who were consistently ruining the schedule.

Early Birds

A number of practices suffer from the opposite problem: patients who regularly come early. One pediatrician had several patients who routinely showed up a half hour early, along with various brothers, sisters, and other family members tagging along. To solve the problem, he had the receptionist screen these patients, letting them know first that they would not be seen before their assigned time. Charts of chronic early patients were coded, and he tried to schedule these patients early in the morning or afternoon, before the reception room became full.

Inadequate Scheduling

Inadequate scheduling usually occurs because the person who takes the appointment does not ask enough questions. It is difficult to schedule a patient for the correct period of time without knowing the purpose of the appointment. There is a vast difference between the time that would be scheduled for the removal of a suture and the time set aside for an annual physical examination. Therefore, it is important for your assistant to screen calls and determine the nature of each problem.

Sometimes a patient may be reluctant to tell the receptionist the reason for the appointment. When patients want to know why your medical assistant is questioning them, they should be told, "The doctor has asked me to determine the nature of the problem so that I can schedule enough time with him for a proper examination." Usually this explanation will lead most patients to indicate why they want the appointment. If a patient is still hesitant about discussing the problem, you might have your assistant schedule him or her for a quick telephone consultation with you during the time you normally make telephone calls.

Time-Consuming Questions and Routines

A number of time-consuming questions can significantly delay your schedule. One family practitioner has all the frequently asked questions on preprinted sheets, which are placed in a wall rack mounted in each examination room. He has 30 information sheets to date; every time he hears another question he thinks he will have to answer again, he dictates a detailed answer so that it can be printed up for the next questioner.

Another approach, used by an ear, nose, and throat specialist, is to use a videotape recorder to record his answers to such questions. He uses the patient education room extensively. Likewise, a nurse can arrange the appropriate presentation for a patient; if she is well trained and qualified, she will be able to do it very well.

A well-thought-out and developed scheduling system is important for maximizing your personal efficiency as well as keeping your patients satisfied. To achieve this, you need to analyze your scheduling problems, and be committed to taking an active role in solving them. As you try to set up a customized appointment scheduling system that reflects the specific needs of your practice, you will be establishing the efficient office systems and procedures necessary to improve the quality of the time you spend with your patients. The following chapter will describe a proved method to survey your schedule, with a view to custom-tailoring a schedule for you. The increased quality of health care delivery will significantly affect patient service, and will overcome your number-one patient objection.

●

Chapter 19

How to Survey Your Schedule

Just as airlines need to know how long it takes to board an aircraft and get the plane ready and out of the airport so it can reach its next destination on time, it is critical in managing a successful appointment schedule that you know how long it takes to prepare patients and move them through your practice so that you can see your other patients on time. Emergencies and a number of mechanical problems have plagued airlines, and yet they do a superb job of consistently getting passengers to and from destinations on time. To develop a successful schedule for your practice, you must know precisely how long it takes you and your staff to see patients for various types of complaints. It is impossible for you to maintain a schedule if you are not fully aware of these time requirements. Scheduling involves making an intelligent estimate of patients' requirements and sticking to it. Time spent now in surveying your schedule will pay off later in maximizing your time and the time and output of your staff.

Setting Up the Patient Survey Sheet

Before you can modify your appointment system you must conduct a survey of your present system and collect data on every visit. Do

Figure **19-1**

Patient Survey

Date: _____ Doctor's Name _____

Visit type: No show ☐
New pt.—consult   ☐
Minor surg.—intermediate visit   ☐
Follow-up—short visit   ☐
Prenatal   ☐
Miscellaneous   ☐
Patient routine   Time

_____   _____
_____   _____
_____   _____
_____   _____

Interruptions   Time In   Time Out

_____   _____   _____
_____   _____   _____

this by designing a patient survey sheet similar to that shown in Figure 19-1.

Categorize Your Patient Visits

You will find that three to five categories, plus one for miscellaneous activities, are sufficient; however, the number will vary according to the variety of procedures you perform. Most doctors presently operate with three patient visit types—10 minutes, 20 minutes, and 30 minutes—based on time slots in their present appointment books. In this case the patient types to be surveyed could be:

1. Short visit
2. Intermediate visit
3. Long visit
4. Miscellaneous

The goal of the survey is to determine how long each type of visit is actually taking.

A busy specialist in obstetrics and gynecology found that the following breakdown met 90 percent of his needs:

1. New patient appointment and consultation
2. Minor office surgery and intermediate office visits

3. Follow-up and short office visits
4. Prenatal visits
5. Miscellaneous

With these time categories, he developed a system that lets him be more consistently punctual.

Determine the Patient Routine

Survey various components in the routine, beginning with the appointment time and finishing when the patient leaves. Typically, as in Figure 19-1, you will include the appointment time, when the patient enters the examination room, and when the nurse and doctor enter and leave the examination room. You can also survey various subcomponents of your routine.

One family practitioner used the survey method to determine the number of blood pressure measurements he was performing and the amount of time spent on them. When he examined the data, he decided that he was spending too much time on these procedures; he began to delegate such duties to a medical assistant and spent his time on more difficult work.

Record Interruptions

Every time an interruption occurs when you are with a patient within the survey period, mark the interruption time in and out. Be conscientious with this, as it will give you a more accurate picture of the various breaks in your schedule. After you have examined the causes of these interruptions, you will be able to deal with them more efficiently.

Administering the Survey

Determine Your Survey Period

To be statistically accurate you should conduct the survey on every patient who comes into your office over a two-month period; however, some practitioners save time and do the survey over an average two-week period. You will have to make a judgment on whether it is an average week, so that you can get a relevant sample. For example, if there is a flu epidemic or if that particular week is an otherwise abnormal one—for example, in midsummer—you should delay the survey and choose a time that you feel adequately represents patient flow in your office.

Survey Every Patient

Have your assistant clip a survey sheet to the medical record of every patient who comes into the office during the survey period. Normally, the medical assistant will enter most of the patient routine on the form. You will enter only the time you went in to see the patient and the time you left, as well as any interruptions that occurred during that time frame.

Sort the Survey Sheets

At the end of the survey period, sort the patient flow sheets by doctor and type of visit. Your goal is to work out averages for the various types of visits to each doctor in the practice. If you have five different types of visits listed, plus a miscellaneous category, you should have six piles. Sort the patient flow sheets by day—you will have consecutive Mondays for one type of visit at the top, and consecutive Tuesdays together, and so on. In this way, you can get an idea on work loads on various days of the week when you do your final survey. When you have completed this procedure, work out the average times.

Summarizing the Data

Figure 19-2 is a patient routine summary, arranged by type of visit; this form is used to summarize the patient survey sheets. The statistics

Figure 19-2

Patient Routine Summary

Visit type:
1. Average time in reception room   _____
2. Average time with nurse   _____
3. Average time with doctor   _____
4. Average patient time waiting in exam room _____
5. Average time from visit completion to patient leaving the office   _____
6. Total average patient time in office   _____
7. Number of visits   _____

| Mon. | Tues. | Wed. | | Thurs. | Fri. | Sat. |

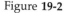

Special Notes:

you gather here will show you how long you take with various types of visits and give you a breakdown of the patient routine by time period. Once you have a good grasp of patients in the office and the time requirements of various routines, you will be ready to assign specific times to your customized schedule.

If your average office call is taking you 12 minutes to complete and you are booking patients into 10-minute time slots, simple arithmetic shows that you will be exactly 60 minutes late by the end of the day, if you schedule 30 patients. Thus, if your appointment schedule really reflected your personal style of practice, you would have 12-minute time slots for office calls in your particular practice.

Appointment books available in stationery stores are only broken into 10-, 15-, and 30-minute time periods. These may be adequate for most business purposes, but when was the last time you completed an office call in exactly 10 or 15 minutes?

Daily Variations

You should also observe how different days of the week vary by visit type. "We didn't need any elaborate survey to tell us that we were consistently late every Monday and Friday," said a busy family practitioner. "I cannot remember a Friday when I was home before 7 P.M.; it seems that many patients drop in or want to be squeezed in on these days because people want to see their doctors before the weekend. Similarly, a lot happens on Saturday and Sunday, making Monday a busier day. We now try to leave more open slots on Mondays and Fridays and seldom book routine visits on these days, anticipating work-ins. We tailored our appointment system to handle the problem."

Your appointment schedule should be designed to reflect daily differences in work patterns. If Monday differs from Tuesday, then your appointment book should reflect that difference. However, consistency is the criterion in a good appointment schedule and your goal should be to set up an appointment system that consistently matches the way your practice operates. You will also have a more precise idea of the various types of visits being performed on various days of the week.

Pinpoint Interruptions

When summarizing your patient flow sheets, compile a summary log of interruptions (Figure 19-3). Only by understanding what

Figure 19-3

Interruptions Summary

Average time

1. Calls from doctors   _____
2. Calls from patients   _____
3. Staff requests   _____
4. Other _____ _____
   _____   _____
   _____   _____

Interruptions by day

Mon.	Tues	Wed.	Thurs.	Fri.	Sat.
____	____	____	____	____	____

Special Notes:

interruptions are destroying your schedule can you begin to control them, rather than having the schedule control you. Try to discern whether interruptions occur more on various days of the week or more at certain times of the day than at others.

Once you get a feel for interruptions, you can then begin to schedule them into your system. For example, if you happen to have frequent calls from physicians on Mondays, you could schedule fewer visits that day than on other days of the week. Another approach is to schedule annual physical examinations on Tuesdays, Wednesdays, and Thursdays, if these are the days when the fewest interruptions occur.

After you have completed your practice survey and have a list of your summaries and interruptions, you can begin to design your own customized appointment schedule. You will also be maximizing your time, which in turn will increase your output and put you in control of your schedule and your life.

Chapter 20

Customized Appointment Schedule: Your Key to Seeing Patients on Time

Have you ever wondered why you use your current appointment scheduling system? For many doctors, it was the free book supplied by the friendly detail person when they first started practice—and they are still using it. Ninety-nine percent of all doctors use either a 15-minute or a 10-minute appointment system. However, as I am sure you will understand as you read on, there really cannot be a standard appointment format for all physicians, since all physicians practice differently. Therefore, a customized schedule is the one that is most appropriate for your office. The customized schedule can be adapted to reflect your individuality and your practice style and specialty. Thus you will be better able to deliver more efficient service, which will pay off by enabling you to see more patients and by promoting your practice as a competent, efficient one.

Remember that everything that involves your time should be on your appointment schedule, including hospital rounds, meetings, surgery, and so on. It is best if this schedule is maintained by only one person in the office (Figure 20-1).

167

Figure 20-1

Appointment Scheduling

Date _____ Day _____

Surgery

Time	Patient	Procedure			Place

In-hospital visits

Place	Patient		Reminders (meetings)

Telephone

Patient							
Type	Time	Last name	First	Chart no.	Day	Night	Reason for visit

No shows		Called and cancelled		Stand-by		
Patient	Time	Patient	Time	Patient	Tele	Note

□ New patient—consult   ○ Follow-up—short visit
△ Minor surgery—intermediate visit

On the left hand side of the schedule shown is a column headed "Type." In this particular example, the various types of appointments are denoted by symbols (you can choose your own method). This allows the appointment secretary to know how many types of openings are left within a certain day. Also note that the time frames for each type of visit are customized from the numbers in the summary of your appointment survey.

If you have an alphabetical filing system, record the patient's surname in the appointment book first, to speed up pulling files. If you have a numerical filing system, include a place on the schedule for the chart number.

When patients call for an appointment, record on the schedule telephone numbers where they can be reached both during the day and in the evening. This is very useful if you have to reschedule patients or call them to remind them of their visits.

There should be a spot for the general reason for each visit. Each patient who calls for an appointment should be asked the reason for the visit. This lets the appointment secretary decide what type of time slot to allocate. All of this information can be recorded very quickly.

Patients who did not show up or who called and canceled their appointments that particular day are listed in the space at the bottom of the sheet. It is a good idea to keep these records for medicolegal purposes.

Note that there is a space for listing patients on standby. When an appointment is unexpectedly canceled, a standby list permits you to call in another patient, thereby ensuring a smooth patient flow with no gaps in the schedule.

The schedule should conform to your practice, and not your practice to the schedule. A customized schedule that reflects how your practice sees patients allows you to make your system more efficient and minimizes your patients' chief complaint about your practice. You will also be using your own time more effectively, allowing you to increase your output and at the same time enhance your practice for your patients.

●

Chapter 21

Patient Information Booklets

A successful practice depends as much on the collective contribution of patients who comply with their treatment as on efficient practice operations. To run a smooth and effective practice for all patients, you need their cooperation. You can gain this cooperation in several ways— through your discussions with patients, and through your staff members' interaction with patients, coupled with constant reinforcement. Patient information booklets specify the policies of your practice and are an inexpensive, subtle public relations tool that reinforce the values and philosophies of the practice in the patients' minds.

Types of Patient Information Booklets

Patient information booklets have two basic objectives. (1) They promote the positive benefits of the practice to the patients; in effect, they are excellent public relations promotional devices that you can use for practice building purposes. (2) Perhaps more important, they describe the functions of your practice, which may include your practice philosophy; in addition, they let patients know how they can cooperate in their own care. Also, the information orients them to the practice and

171

to the way that your particular systems and procedures affect them. Many times a delicate policy (for example, one that calls for payment at the time of service) can be explained better in a booklet than orally. The patient information booklet also lets the patient know how your practice operates from the patient's point of view. In addition to dealing with your philosophy of practice, it describes your credentials and your organization.

Some practices have two brochures—one for public relations purposes, which does not discuss any of the financial systems, collection procedures, and other patient compliance issues. The second booklet, which could be titled *The Patient Handbook,* details all the patient compliance issues. Thus, one booklet would be used strictly for promotional purposes to potential new patients, and the second would be used as a handbook that they would receive when entering the practice. Most practices, however, combine both of these objectives in one comprehensive publication. Whichever approach you choose, you will need a balance of both public relations and patient compliance issues to make this publication successful.

Benefits of Patient Information Booklets

1. Patient information booklets are an excellent, ethical public relations tool that can present the practice in the best possible light.
2. They are an efficient way of communicating your philosophy of practice and providing patient orientation.
3. They can serve as a good basis for orienting new patients to your practice.
4. Patients keep the brochure and show their friends, so that it can be an excellent practice building tool.
5. They introduce a uniform, organized approach to patient handling in your practice.
6. They steer patient communication around a written record, thus reducing potential interpersonal conflicts between patients and staff.
7. They encourage you and your staff to reevaluate your practice policies and procedures since you will be communicating these to your patients.
8. They offer an excellent way to dovetail your current systems and procedures so that patients know how things are done and why.

9. They tell patients what is expected of them when they visit your office, and therefore help prevent misunderstandings about your office procedures.

10. They can reduce telephone calls by as much as 30 percent. When you consider that the average primary care practice receives about 100 calls per day, a savings of 30 percent, or 30 calls at two minutes per call, can save as much as one hour of a receptionist's time per day.

Welcoming Your Patient

A "hello" or "welcome" message from you to your patients is a good way to begin. Include some information about the following in this introduction: (1) the history of your practice, (2) your practice organization, (3) the philosophy of your practice, (4) a short description of your specialty, (5) a description of your background, and (6) the purpose of the book.

The tone should be established by using the word "we," addressing the patients as members of the overall practice team. An example of this approach is as follows:

> Welcome to our practice. The purpose of this booklet is to help us work together toward the improvement of your health. Each patient whom we have the privilege to serve is entitled to, and will receive, the best care we can provide. Together we will work as a team in achieving the common goal of providing the quality care you deserve.

You should also include specific information about yourself—the year you graduated from medical school, your additional training, and your specific philosophy of medicine, as well as an overall description of how you practice.

Spell Out Your Appointment Policies

Appointment procedures should be clearly spelled out for your patients. The booklet should tell your patients how far in advance they have to schedule various types of appointments, your cancellation policy (and whether you charge for broken appointments), how appointments are made, and what your policy is for work-ins and walk-ins.

It is good to mention the negative effects caused by patients who are continually late or constantly break their appointments. If your medical assistant has been instructed to ask for the nature of the problem when patients call for appointments, let your patients know why she is doing it; patients will then be more willing to answer the questions honestly. The booklet should explain the request as allowing the doctor to "schedule enough time together to care for your problem adequately." Details about office hours, closing days, and how appointments are handled during off hours should also be included. Finally, remind your patients about the importance of being on time. Explain why you will sometimes be behind in your schedule. When patients better understand your problems they will be more sympathetic when you are delayed.

Detail Your Telephone Policies

Your patient information booklet should describe your policies about the use of the telephone, which is truly the lifeline to your practice. Patients who understand your telephone procedures—why things are done in certain ways—will be far more sympathetic when problems occur, and also know how the system works. One busy family practitioner encourages patients to call about appointments and nonurgent matters during slack telephone hours; in his practice, peak hours are between 11 A.M. and 2 P.M. and from 3 P.M. to 4 P.M. Patients know that if they call during nonpeak hours they will experience fewer delays getting through to him.

The booklet should state whether you charge for telephone advice and under what circumstances you do this. Some physicians do not believe in dispensing medical advice over the telephone. If this is your policy, say so, possibly with the explanation: "Many illnesses have similar symptoms, so if you have developed a complication or new problem, please understand the need for an examination in our office, rather than discussions over the telephone."

Remember to give your patients the reasons why you have decided on a certain policy. If you have designated times for returning calls, let the patients know what these times are. Encourage patients who are calling long distance to call during the time you normally make call-backs. These sessions should be scheduled at the same time every day. I recommend that you make call-backs two or three times a day (and perhaps as many as four)—once in midmorning, once in midafternoon, and again at the end of the day.

Your policy on the communication of laboratory test results can be handled in the telephone management section of your patient information brochure. It is also important to include your policy on prescription renewals; suggest to your patients that they have the telephone number of the pharmacy and the prescription number on hand before they call you. You might add the following cautions:

> We are very reluctant to renew prescriptions for tranquilizers or sleeping pills, as they are only a short-term solution and in the long term can only compound the patient's problems.
>
> For renewal of antibiotics, such as penicillin, we would appreciate your seeing the doctor. This will allow him to assess your progress before adding more medication, so that you only take as much as your illness warrants.

Spell Out Your Billing and Insurance Processing Policy

If you participate in local insurance plans—that is, accept payment directly from the insurer—it is a good idea to explain the procedure in your brochure.

I also recommend that you list your most common fees on a separate insert sheet in the patient information booklet for your patients, because this information might have to be changed two or three times a year, depending on market forces and the economic situation of your practice. If you expect payment at the time of service for all fees under $25, that should be stated. You should also describe how your office handles delinquent accounts. If you have one person in charge of billing and collections, let your patients know who this is, and state whether you charge for completing insurance forms.

Other Helpful Information

Consider sending a stack of patient information booklets to your referring physicians; make sure they include maps that tell how to reach your office. Alternatively, your office could mail these to patients before their scheduled visit.

A section entitled Other Helpful Information can include mention of the no-smoking policy in your practice, if applicable. It can also include your policy with respect to the transfer of medical records; the confidentiality of the medical record should be stressed.

Let Your Patients Know What a Good Patient Is

A section entitled How You Can Help lets your patients know what you expect from them and what it takes to become an ideal patient; this can help them move toward that goal. Some of the things you might like to consider would include the following:

1. Always telephone for appointments in advance.
2. If you are unable to keep an appointment, please let us know—as far in advance as possible.
3. Every time you come into the office please let the receptionist know of any changes in address, telephone number, marital status, or insurance information.
4. Check your charges before you leave the office. If you have any questions, feel free to ask the receptionist at the desk.
5. Check your bill carefully when you receive it. Call the office about any errors, so that they can be corrected.
6. All patients under 18 must have written parental permission for treatment.
7. If you have any complaints, please put them in writing to help us correct them. These may be mailed or left with the patient relations coordinator.
8. We welcome any suggestions you have.

Miscellaneous Policy Areas to Address

You need to describe your policies and communicate them to your patients concisely. You should let your patients know under what circumstances you would refer them for consultations and that you try to make it easy for them to obtain a second opinion. Your brochure should also communicate your policy on laboratory and x-ray reports. Here is the wording from one practice's booklet:

> Tests that are to be reported to you by telephone rather than by return appointment will be done by physicians who are familiar with your problem after the tests have been completed. Patients need not call the office for reports. If the office has not called you within five working days, the tests have come back and everything is fine.

Launching the Booklet

All of your assistants should be involved in developing a practice profile as a first step to writing the booklet. Different staff members should describe the practice from their own points of view. The receptionist, for example, can discuss her recurring problems, and the billing clerk should list her recommendations about billing disputes. You could delegate the whole project to a medical assistant who has some talent and writing ability. Often the process of putting together a booklet forces staff members and physicians to discuss lingering problem areas.

After the practice profile is finished, hold a brainstorming session with the whole staff. Your assistants should come to the meeting with their own lists of things to be included in the booklet, and the meeting should elaborate on these ideas. The total staff involvement will build staff interest in the project and better contribute to the implementation and final success of the booklet.

The tone of the booklet and how it is written is very important. It should be written for the patient in an inclusive tone, using the word "we," rather than implying that these are the "rules and regulations" of the practice. It should bring home the point that the patient, staff, and physician are all on the same team, working together to improve patient care and staff efficiency.

Once the booklet is written and edited, have it typed using a high-quality typewriter. Consider having an art student illustrate it. An 8 ½ × 11 inch, three-fold brochure is the least expensive method to use. You may consider folding two 8 ½ × 11 inch sheets in two halves, one sheet inside the other, and stapling them in the middle. Both these methods are inexpensive, and it will cost about $100 to $500 to print 2,000 booklets on high-quality paper.

After a six-month trial period, review the booklet and correct any problems that have emerged. After correction and approval of the revision, you should consider having the booklet professionally typeset and printed. The booklet should be given to new patients as they come into your practice; you should also consider mailing one to each family currently associated with your practice. It is best if the physician hands the booklet to the patient; however, if this cannot be done, it is acceptable for the medical assistant to do it. Reinforce the purpose and use of the booklet by saying something like this: "Here is the patient information booklet we have prepared to help us serve you better. Please read it, keep it, and refer to it." In referral practice, mail the booklet to the patient before he or she arrives for the first visit.

To ensure that the patient will keep the book, consider leaving a space for the patient's name, blood type, drug allergies, immunization history, and other general medical information. If there is medically oriented information about the patient in the booklet, he or she will be more likely to keep it. It is important to reinforce what the booklet says to make it a success. With new patients, take the time on the first visit to go over the information. After the initial briefing, every time a patient asks a routine question that is answered in print, always refer the patient back to the booklet. When patients get used to using the information, you will find that your practice will begin to run very smoothly.

Once your patient information booklet has been launched and reinforced in your patient's mind, it will become a valuable tool to give you greater control over patient management and to help eliminate the patient-practice communication gap. For effective patient service, you will need good team work between patients, medical assistants, and physicians. You must remember, too, that the patient is an equal partner in the team that delivers health care to your patients. In that regard, like an employee, the patient needs to be oriented to what a good patient does and is. The more precise your communication, the better the final results will be with patients, and the greater your overall practice satisfaction.

Keep in mind the difference between a patient promotion booklet and a patient compliance booklet. When writing the book, consider carefully whether you are looking at patient compliance issues or promotional issues. Although both can be mixed in the booklet, I strongly suggest that you separate them. The patient promotional book should be used to emphasize the benefits and positive features of the practice. The patient compliance booklet should be given to your own patients for their orientation to the practice. Patient information booklets are a key step to a well-run and patient-oriented practice. Use them well and effectively, and your patients will appreciate you and your practice even more.

Chapter 22

The Telephone: Lifeline to Your Practice

The telephone, as noted earlier, is your lifeline—the primary channel of communication between you and your patients. Patients' impressions of you and your practice are largely determined by the effective use of excellent telephone technique. Since you never have a second chance at a first impression, your medical assistant must understand and always use good telephone manners. Excellent telephone skills are easy, cost-effective ways of marketing your practice as a warm, competent one.

An effective telephone communication system is only possible if your receptionist follows written telephone systems and procedures and if you obtain good telephone equipment. Therefore, your patient relations coordinators should be well trained in the use of excellent telephone technique. They should have an understanding of why the telephone is important in establishing your practice as a responsive, efficient one. Consider the positive impression projected by a warm and caring receptionist as she communicates with your patients on the telephone.

Project Consistency of Service—Answer Within Three Rings

Studies show that callers are most receptive to the party answering if the response comes within three rings. Beyond that, callers tend to become perturbed and unreceptive. Furthermore, answering quickly helps to create an impression of efficiency in the patients' minds, and they begin to respect their physician's office systems. As consumers come to expect high levels of service from many contacts in their daily environment, they begin to expect the same high level of service from you and your practice. Physicians who realize this stand to reap significant benefits.

Portray the Warmth and Understanding You Have

Patients appreciate warmth and understanding in their dealings with all members of your staff. By having the receptionist first identify the office, then introduce herself, and then offer assistance, an image is projected that yours is a warm, friendly practice, with a "real" person answering the telephone who is able and eager to give assistance.

Such small but important techniques as explaining why the doctor can not come to the telephone are simply common courtesy. Be sure to have your assistant let the caller know that the doctor is unavailable before asking for identification. Otherwise, you may very well have a disgruntled caller who feels discriminated against or brushed aside.

Use the caller's name as frequently as possible. This may seem unimportant at first, but studies have shown that people warm up instantly to someone who uses their name in the course of a conversation. Try this technique yourself and train your assistant to use the same approach to reap the warm and positive responses from your happy patients.

Let Your Patients Know What They Can Expect

Establishing when the call will be returned sets patients' minds at ease. It lets them plan to be home when the call comes and keep the line free. The following is an example of good telephone protocol:

Ring . . . Ring . . .
Receptionist: "Good morning. Dr. Bell's office. Sally speaking. May I help you?"

Caller: "May I speak with Dr. Bell?"

R.: "Dr. Bell is with a patient right now. May I ask who's calling?"

C.: "Yes. This is Mrs. George Smith from Maple Drive."

R.: "Yes, Mrs. Smith—May I help you?"

C.: "My son has a temperature of 104°; I'd really like to talk with the doctor."

R.: "I'm sorry to hear that, Mrs. Smith. I'll report this to doctor and have him call you. Dr. Bell usually makes his call-backs between 1 and 2 o'clock. Is that a convenient time for you?"

C.: "Yes. I'll make it a point to keep the line free at that time."

R.: "Thank you for calling, Mrs. Smith." (Hangs up gently.)

The following is a summary of what your receptionist ought to be doing routinely.

1. Answer the telephone within three rings 90 percent of the time.
2. Identify the practice by name—for example, "Dr. Smith's office."
3. Identify herself—for example, "Linda speaking."
4. Offer assistance—"May I help you?"
5. If the doctor can't come to the phone immediately, give the reason—"Dr. Smith is with a patient right now."
6. Ask for the caller's name early in the conversation: "May I ask who's calling?"
7. Use the caller's name whenever possible during the conversation.
8. Determine early the nature of the call.
9. Establish a priority on whether the call needs to be:
   a. Put through right away.
   b. Returned later this morning—or later in the week.
10. Ask, "Is there anything I can do?" or suggest, "Perhaps I can help you."
11. Inform the caller when to expect a return call—"Dr. Smith usually makes his call-backs between 1:00 and 2:00 P.M. Is that convenient for you?"

Improve Your Receptionist's "Smileability"

It is the intangible aspects of handling the telephone that truly distinguish the good receptionist from the excellent receptionist. Does she actually smile when she picks up the receiver? You can usually sense a warm individual by voice intonation. A person who smiles while talking presents a friendlier image of your practice. Also, an interesting, pleasant voice can have a tremendous impact. One doctor installed mirrors near the telephone so the staff could see themselves and improve their "smileability."

The following is a list of key ingredients that improve the telephone personality of your practice.

1. The receptionist should actually smile when she identifies the office.
2. She should speak directly into the mouthpiece, with her mouth one inch away from it.
3. She should speak clearly and distinctly.
4. She should vary the pitch of her voice and speed of delivery.
5. She should present a positive attitude and helpful approach.
6. She should speak grammatically.
7. Her voice should be expressive.

You have a right to expect that your receptionist will exhibit your caring philosophy by maintaining this high quality of telephone technique.

Handle Each Call With Careful Consideration

Patients feel the most aggravated at being put on hold without being given any other option when they call a doctor's office. The receptionist should be aware that the person on the line may be calling from a distance and it may be cheaper or preferable for him or her to call back rather than stay on hold. Callers should always be asked whether they mind waiting before they are put on hold. It is common courtesy to give your patients a choice. Nine out of 10 callers will agree to be put on hold. Assuming they do agree, your receptionist should check back every couple of minutes to assure callers that they have not been forgotten and to determine whether they still wish to remain on hold.

When on the telephone, both you and your receptionist should give the caller your full attention. Carrying on a conversation with someone else while you are on the telephone can be considered nothing but rude. It is also important to follow each call to its logical conclusion so that the caller feels satisfied. For example, a patient may require some information regarding a prescription renewal or a billing document; this inquiry should be followed through to the patient's satisfaction.

The following are some key considerations in handling calls.

1. Always ask callers if they mind holding, and wait for their reply before putting them on hold.

2. Check every minute or two with people on hold to let them know they have not been forgotten.

3. Give the caller your full attention, and never carry on a conversation with someone else while handling a telephone call.

4. When the call is completed, always allow the caller to hang up first.

5. At the call's completion, end the conversation by thanking the caller for calling.

6. Hang up gently.

7. Do not ask who the caller is before saying the doctor is not available.

8. Tell the doctor who is on the line before transferring the call.

9. Follow through every call to its logical conclusion.

10. Know where the doctor is at all times in case it is necessary to reach him.

Figure **22-1.** Call-handling protocol.

Doctor will take the following calls immediately:

1. Any patient with any of the following symptoms:
   —severe pain
   —heavy bleeding
   —in shock—going unconscious
2. Other physician
3. Other patients first screened by nursing
4. Hospitals regarding patient progress
5. Immediate family

Doctor will call back:
1. Patients screented by nursing
2. Management consultant
3. Accountant
4. Lawyer
5. Medical society
6. Friends

Nursing will take the following calls:
1. New patient who wants to talk with the doctor
2. Patient with questions about current treatment
3. Pharmacy
4. Patient wanting prescription renewed
5. Laboratory
6. Patient about laboratory result

Administrative assistant will take all other administrative calls.

Figure 22-2. Sample of a message form.

Urgency No. 1 _____ **No. 2** _____ **No. 3** _____	

For _____
(doctor, nurse, asst.)

M _____ No. _____
Patient's full name   Chart no.

(   )- _____   (   )- _____
Tel. no. home   Tel. no. work

☐ Fever _____ — _____
Temperature   How long

☐ Chest _____—_____—_____
pain   Where   Intensity   How long

☐ RX   _____ — _____
refill   RX no.   Pharmacy tel no.
_____
Drug

☐ Miscellaneous _____

Please call by:
☐ _____ A.M./P.M.
☐ Returned your call
☐ Telephoned
☐ Wants an earlier
     appointment
☐ Will call back

Message _____
_____
_____
_____
_____
_____
_____

Disposition

Date: _____ Time: _____ A.M./P.M.

By _____ By _____ By _____
      taken by   action taken   recorded

Call type
   A1,A2,A3,A4,B,D1,D2,L,NP,NPA,O,P,   Misc. _____

Emergency Call Handling

A call-handling protocol should be established to handle all emergencies. Figure 22-1 is an example of such a protocol. The message pad (Figure 22-2) should also be customized to obtain useful information for disposition. For management purposes you can summarize the type of calls on the end-of-day summary (Figure 22-3).

Before you actually take the call, your message pad should be completely filled out, the medical records should be pulled, and either

Figure 22-3

```
┌─────────────────────────────────────────────────────────────────────────┐
│  End of Day Summary                                                       │
│                                                                           │
│                                                                           │
│  A1—Make an appointment        _____   A4  —Misc. reappoinment   _____  │
│  A2—Cancel an appointment      _____   B   —Billing              _____  │
│  A3—Reschedule an appointment  _____   D1  —Doctor               _____  │
│                                                                           │
│  D2—Pt. for doctor             _____   NPA—New ptnt. appointment  _____ │
│  L —Lab. results               _____   O   —Office management    _____  │
│  NP—New pt. inquiry            _____   P   —Prescription         _____  │
│  Misc. (specify) _____│
│  Total Calls _____                                    │
└─────────────────────────────────────────────────────────────────────────┘
```

the patient relations coordinator or the clinical coordinator should have obtained triage information from the patient.

Handle Your Calls Pleasantly and Efficiently

To make the best use of your time on the telephone, you should schedule your call-backs at regularly designated times, rather than fit them in on a casual basis. This will fulfill your calling obligation, and will allow you to concentrate on the patients in your office. It also lets you prepare for the call so as to keep it as much to the point as possible.

If your receptionist places a call for you ahead of time and gets the patient on the line first, you will save a few precious minutes each day. Insist that telephone messages passed on to you be detailed enough so that the degree of urgency of the medical problem is clear. Have your assistant pull the charts of the patients receiving the call-backs.

Use Quality Equipment

To make the most of your telephone's potential, you need good equipment to complement your office's courtesy and efficiency. In today's competitive environment callers should not find your office's line busy. Therefore, you should consider asking your local telephone company for a *busy signal study* and a *peak load study*. A busy signal study tells you how many times people call your office and find the line busy, and a peak load study shows when people have called, so that you will know the times at which the majority of your calls are coming in. This will help you determine if you need more telephone lines. The studies are free in many situations.

Another nice touch for your reception room would be to have a telephone for the use of your patients, so that they could make calls from your practice. The telephone should either be controlled from behind the reception desk or have a long-distance call stopper on it. One useful piece of equipment for your phone is a chime instead of the usual harsh telephone ring. It is more pleasant for you as well as for your patients, and it creates a very positive atmosphere.

The following considerations should help you decide about the equipment that your practice should have in place.

1. Make available two incoming lines and one outgoing line per doctor.
2. Consider a direct line to the pharmacy.
3. Consider a direct line to the admitting department of the hospital.
4. Make available a telephone for patients, so they do not ask to make calls from the reception desk.
5. Install push-button telephones.
6. Install an automatic dialing feature for frequently made calls.
7. Install a privacy feature to block out anyone listening in on your conversation.
8. Your telephone equipment should allow you to dictate over the telephone when your office is closed.
9. Your telephone equipment should alow your receptionist to signal ahead who is on the line.
10. All telephones in the office should be wall mounted.
11. Have your receptionist use a headset rather than the conventional receiver.
12. Replace the conventional ring with a chime, and provide music for callers on hold.
13. Have a pen attached to or near each telephone.
14. Have a busy signal study conducted to determine if more than 10 percent of your callers are being turned away.
15. Have a peak load study conducted to find out your peak times for telephone calls.

Project Confidence—Organize the Call for Efficiency

Organized systems and procedures project the image that your office is efficient. Specific systems and procedures help in creating a tight telephone system. You should establish how each telephone call will be answered, handled, and followed through. To do this effectively, you need to have a number of systems in place, including telephone logs and a customized message pad. Listed below in summary form are the key items that should be addressed in your systems and procedures:

1. Every call should be noted in a telephone log.
2. A customized message pad should be beside the telephone at all times to record the required patient information.
3. Each message should be taken in duplicate, using carbon paper, to ensure that every call is logged.
4. Names of all patients who call and cancel their appointments should be noted in the log and in their charts (for medicolegal reasons).
5. Names of all patients who fail to keep their appointments should be noted in their charts.
6. A detailed message should be taken for every call-back.
7. Each telephone message should be disposed of in the chart.
8. Office staff should be familiar with the procedure for an emergency.
9. Office staff should have a list of emergency symptoms.
10. A list of frequently called numbers should be at hand.
11. Staff members' personal calls should be kept to a minimum.
12. Ascertain that after-hours answering service is adequate.
13. Make sure a log is kept of all outgoing long distance calls.
14. Provide a written call handling protocol system for the benefit of your staff.

Mastering the telephone skills required in a medical office means more than possessing an agile finger and a silver tongue. It requires a naturally positive person, who is perceptive of people's needs and trained in the use of good telephone techniques; such a person has a favorable effect on the image your practice presents to the public. To maximize your telephone's value, your staff members need to know how to use the telephone as a good public relations device. This can be accomplished through the establishment of good written telephone procedures, which must be adhered to at all times, according to the highest standard of excellence.

Sometimes we regard the telephone as a necessary nuisance that must be tolerated in modern-day living. But, like any other invention, it is how we use it that counts. Train your staff to use the telephone with respect, and you will be taking an active step towards increased practice growth.

●

Chapter 23

Medical Records Management

To maintain a strong and thriving practice, it is critical that you have an effective and well-designed medical records and filing management system. There are two basic aspects to an effective records management system: (1) the actual organization of the record, including the way that you capture data on the record (whether by means of dictation, checklists, or writing), and the efficient retrieval of information from that record, and (2) a well-thought-out filing system that minimizes time in pulling and retrieving files, as well as eliminating misfiled records. An effective and well-thought-out system not only improves your ability to deliver quality care to your patients, it is also the heart of the practice and allows you to provide efficient and effective medical care.

Misfiled records can be extremely costly in terms of staff time, and there can be dire consequences to the patient as a result of these errors. If you or your staff are unable to find a record, it tends to diminish confidence in your practice and your service. The cost of a misfiled record is higher than you might think, since it includes not only the time taken to find the misfiled records, but also the risk of potential liability in not having the chart, as well as the lost goodwill.

When a patient sits in your office watching you shuffle among the pages of his or her record for two or three minutes trying to find the progress report from the previous visit, the patient will lose confidence in you and think of you as disorganized. Doctors who read the charts in front of their patients also have difficulty achieving rapport with the patients—it is better to have the correct information ready before the patient comes into the office. Inefficient management of medical records leads to a deterioration of practice efficiency and the delivery of effective medical care, in addition to diminishing patient confidence in the practice. Effective medical records management has the following advantages:

1. If the record is completely organized in a systematic fashion and tailored around the way you like to work, the most important information you want should be instantly readable and accessible to you to maximize your time.

2. Efficient recording decreases your chances for malpractice suits by making crucial information obvious. For example, it is less likely that you will prescribe a drug to which a patient is allergic if the information is located in an obvious and prominent spot on the chart rather than placed in disorganized fashion in some obscure place.

3. Efficient filing saves expensive staff time and frees them to give more attention to handling patients. According to my statistics, staff salaries account for 15 to 18 percent of gross practice revenues (and approximately 50 percent of the cost of filing is in staff time). With conventional filing systems, much of the time is spent in opening and closing drawers, and in filing and retrieving records. By reducing filing time through the use of the newer methods, your practice can save time and money.

4. Efficient filing aids you in billing. If your record clearly and concisely shows what was accomplished with the patient, your nurses or billing clerk can easily pull out this information for billing purposes. Often, procedures that you have carried out are missed because of poor charting techniques, and this can cost you a significant amount over a practice career.

5. Space can be used more efficiently when filing is well organized. Our client statistics indicate that rent accounts for about seven percent of gross practice expenses. Since four-drawer filing cabinets take up to 50 percent more space than open shelf lateral files, this wasted space can be used more effectively for other purposes. A new physician opening his practice currently can save in the neighborhood of $10,000 in rent over a practice career by reducing the space needed by the newer filing systems.

6. As already discussed, misplaced records are expensive. By having a system in place that eliminates misplaced records or spots them easily, you will not only save valuable staff time but also increase patient rapport with your practice.

7. Quality assurance in the medical practice is increased through effective filing systems. With greater emphasis on price competition and the involvement of new delivery systems, an efficient filing system will capture the data necessary for quality assurance in your practice.

Make Optimal Use of Each Medical Record

There are a number of rules and guidelines that should be considered in the tailoring of a useful working system. Each medical record should be more than just a repository for an accumulation of data—it should actually work for you and your patient. If your system is neat, clear, and concise, that will enable you to read your records faster and minimize your chances of making errors. If you can locate and read previous instructions to patients, you can quickly ask them about the results, thus improving patient compliance. Information should be legible, which is easier if you use preprinted stamps and forms where possible.

If your handwriting is difficult to read, you might take one of the courses that offer handwriting improvement instructions specifically for physicians. One such course advertised, "Your handwriting may be dangerous to your wealth," referring to a recent court decision where a physician lost a malpractice case because he was unable to decipher exactly what he had written in a patient's chart.

Physicians in high-volume practices should be strongly encouraged to dictate their medical records rather than write them. This is based on a very simple economic principle—the average person speaks 80 to 100 words a minute, while handwriting is done at a speed of about 20 words per minute. Consequently, the efficiency of physicians can be greatly improved through dictating their notes. Your time is probably worth about $80 per hour, while a secretary's time is worth $8 per hour. Thus, your dictation becomes cost-effective when one hour of transcription can save you more than six minutes of time.

If you choose to dictate your records, you should avoid leaving all dictation to the end of the day. It then becomes an arduous task that rarely gets done. You should consider the patient visit completed only after you have done the dictation. A number of physicians dictate directly in front of the patient, but this is an individual professional decision based on the nature of the case.

Pressure-sensitive (peel-off) paper which can be used for transcription, saves considerable staff time in this process. Continuous-form, precut, pressure-sensitive peel-off paper can be purchased. Most transcription process time is taken in threading the typewriter and setting up the new note, and then taking the paper out of the typewriter and replacing it in the chart. With pressure-sensitive paper, a continuous sheet can be put into the typewriter, and all the notes can be typed onto it. When all the transcription has been completed, the medical assistant only needs to pull off the paper, which has an adhesive backing, and stick it into the appropriate section in the chart. The small cost of the paper saves a great deal of staff time.

Organize the Content

Your personal organization and patient management can be greatly influenced by the use of a well-organized format. Quick location of pertinent information is essential in making the best decision for your patients and the best use of your time. Here are some organizational suggestions derived from physicians all over this country; these ideas can make your charts better for you and your patients.

Consider *tabs* to organize information in the file chart. Some physicians utilize tab systems in their charts to assist in internal file organization. Since physician time is expensive, the well-organized file chart can save money in trying to get information out of charts. One family doctor uses the following organization for his internal tabs:

— TAB A. Data base 1
— TAB B. Data base 2
— TAB C. Progress notes
— TAB D. Lab/x-ray reports/EKG
— TAB E. Problem list
— TAB F. Medications
— TAB G. Miscellaneous

When using tabs, you are balancing the additional cost of the tab with the time the physician saves in trying to get needed information out of the chart.

Consider purchasing *rubber stamps* adapted to your specialty. They are easy to read and are good time savers. There are economical sources of rubber stamps that have a diagram of specific body parts. Other stamps can list specific areas for consideration—for example, WT., HT., B.P., and so on. You may want to choose some stamps of different colors. A red date stamp might denote an injection, or it could denote a follow-up on previous treatment. This allows data to be more easily retrieved from the chart.

Some physicians use *fluorescent stickers* for serious allergies or diseases. Many times these are affixed to the end tab of the record in case they need to be pulled out by the medical assistant.

Utilize the *chart folder* as an important part of the medical record. One doctor lists all diagnoses on the back inside cover, for a quick patient history. Another attaches a memo sheet to the front of the folder, to remind him of what he wants to do or say next time the patient comes in. This is a good place for you to plan to say thank you for patient referrals.

Consider marking the inside of the file folders for *tardy* or *no show patients*, using a T, or an NS. Also consider using color coding for easy identification (preferably this should be on the outside cover of the chart so the medical assistant can see it). This will aid in scheduling your patients for the day, as well as assist you in the event of a malpractice situation. It is critical that all patients who do not appear for appointments be entered in the medical record.

Keep *social progress notes* in an easy place to read in the medical record. This is not taught in medical school, but it is an excellent practice builder that shows your patients how much you care about them. For instance, if there is a death or a birth in a family, your medical assistant might clip the announcement from the newspaper and place it in the file. If the patient is going on a special vacation, you might inquire about his or her destination and make a note in the chart. Next time that patient is in your office, you will amaze him or her with your interest, powerful memory, and sharp observation; it is always worth having this information close at hand.

Good organization of your chart for information purposes is critical to the effective doctor-patient relationship. In order for you to have this information, however, the system should be clearly laid out, so that the pulling and retrieving of records is efficient. After all, anyone can *file* a record; the trick is to *find* it.

Improve Efficiency, Cut Costs

Open shelf filing saves rental space. Open shelf lateral filing can be compared to a bookshelf—rather than a four-drawer file cabinet to house the files, you will have an open shelf system where files are lined up one beside the other on an open shelf, in full view. If desired, a unit can be purchased with lockable doors that pull over the front. Typically, there are five to eight shelves per unit to hold the files. The name of the patient and file number appear on an end tab, which can be easily scanned, the way you might scan the title on the spine of a book. Since files which are housed this way can be stacked two to three feet higher than the four-drawer cabinet, and require no special drawer, space is saved. Furthermore, more space will be available, since you will not need to leave room for opening the drawer to retrieve the files.

Custom build the shelves. Many practices have areas in the office that would be ideal for medical record storage, but not large enough to place a filing unit in. Many practitioners, rather than purchase a standard metal filing system, have carpenters custom build shelves. Since floor space in a business office is at a premium, often the cabinets can be placed in such a way that floor space is not needed. Some practitioners build a filing cabinet into the wall, using the six or eight inches of wall space as filing shelves. The filing cabinet should be within easy reach of the medical assistant.

Use 8½ × 11-inch folders. Although we are beginning a conversion to the metric system, we still live in an 8½ × 11 inch world. Most business stationery and forms still come in that size and you will find that smaller files will cause problems for the file clerk, especially with outside forms and correspondence. Although you may be saving space with small files, the actual cost of customizing internal records and forms can often exceed the cost of the larger 8½ × 11 inch system.

Use *section dividers,* which save the medical assistant's time. A section divider is a thick cardboard or plastic file divider, with an end tab or top tab that marks the beginning of a section. If you are filing alphabetically, you will probably have three to five section dividers per letter of the alphabet. Section dividers, which cost about 20 cents each, serve to single out those areas in which the largest number of files are situated. For example, if you have 20 to 30 patients with the last name of Johnson, you could have a special section divider for the last name. Thus you will be limiting the file search for "Johnson" by going straight to a section divider. Naturally, the section dividers should be customized to the alphabetic or numeric breakdown of patient charts in your practice.

If records are color coded, you can virtually eliminate misplaced records and save considerable staff time. It is an inexpensive technique used to limit the file search. In most systems, 10 basic colors are used. For example, you can affix a half-inch red band to the tab of all the A files. Next, assign another color to all the Bs, and so on, until each of the 10 colors is used and you begin again with red. Most offices will code the charts by the first two letters of the patient's last name, or according to the entire chart number. Consider the name Johnson as an example. Assume that the color blue represents the letter J and yellow represents the letter O. Johnson's chart, therefore, will have two colors: blue and yellow. If Johnson's chart is mistakenly filed under B, the blue color band will be easily seen among the B color bands.

Some physicians doing research add additional colors to the chart identifying various patients with particular symptoms, or patients who are being monitored. Also, file jackets can be purchased in various colors; this can assist you in trying to zero in on specific types of patients.

You can also use *out-guides,* which save staff time. An out-guide is a larger colored file, usually of thicker cardboard or plastic, which is colored yellow or blue for easy recognition. When a medical record is pulled off the shelf, an out-guide can be inserted into the file's place. When the medical assistant refiles the chart, she can zero in on the general area of the file and then look for the out-guide.

Plastic pockets and a *log* can be used in the out-guide to improve the paper flow management and assist in locating charts when they are needed. Letters, reports, and miscellaneous papers can be filed in the out-guide on a daily basis. In this manner, the general refiling of reports will not be disrupted if the file is not on the shelf. Out-guides can be purchased with a preprinted log. On this log, the medical assistant can write the date the file was pulled, and where it is located. This allows you more control over the file, and an audit trail can be established to hunt down the file if it is needed for an emergency.

Fasteners and *plastic pockets* can be permanently attached to the medical record, which assists in organization and eliminates the possibility that loose papers can fall out of the medical record. Paper fasteners can be purchased for about five cents each; one can also obtain small plastic pockets with adhesive backing, which can be permanently affixed to file charts. Fasteners will be used to attach the progress notes and letters to the chart permanently. The small plastic pocket can be used to hold any patient registration cards or small pieces of paper that are needed in the chart.

The decision between *alphabetical* and *numerical systems* is the subject of great debate among medical records filing experts. The main complaint against numerical systems is that the medical assistant has to go to an alphabetical cross-reference to get the patient's number before the chart can be pulled. The key advantage of numerical systems is that they allow faster refiling, and that each person in the practice has a unique number. Ninety percent of all physicians today use alphabetical systems. As a rule of thumb, you should begin to consider a numerical system once you have more than 3,000 active medical charts. The numerical system is more highly organized; if you like everything in your practice to have its proper place, a numerical system might be for you.

Pull inactive charts. It saves valuable office space and staff time to move inactive charts out of your office. Generally, if a patient has not been in to see you within five years, you should pull the chart from your active files and put it in a low-cost storage area. Your initial culling process should be done over a weekend, to minimize office disruption. To make the process easier in the future, a color-coded dot can be affixed to each file when the patient visits your practice in any given year. For example: Assume that a red dot denotes 1979, a yellow dot 1980, and a blue dot 1981. When a patient visits your practice in 1980, put a yellow dot on his chart. If the same patient comes in again, the yellow dot indicates that the patient was seen in 1980, and similarly the red dot indicates the patient was seen in 1979. In 1981, if the same patient comes in again, put a blue dot on the patient chart. Thus, when the time comes to cull the chart, you will know which patients haven't been in for the past five years by noting the colored dots. Make sure all staff members know the color dot code by year. This can be achieved by the use of date stamping.

The inactive charts should be filed alphabetically in the low-cost storage area. Some practices microfilm all inactive charts rather than save the actual paper. With new technology, microfilming costs have decreased significantly.

One can save valuable space by keeping *unnecessary paper* out of the chart. Many practices, rather than saving laboratory reports and consultation letters, summarize the results on flow sheets. The summary can be made by the nurse and checked by the physician as each entry is made. Through the use of flow sheets, files are kept thin and information is made available to the physician at a glance, saving time that would have been spent in flipping through many pages of unneeded information in the charts.

Files for transient or short-term patients are not always necessary. Setting up a new chart on a patient is costly in both filing supplies and staff time. Some practices, rather than open a new chart on every patient, open temporary files for patients seen intermittently in the emergency room or outpatient clinic of a hospital. If the patient is not expected to make a return visit, the physician may consider not opening a chart at all.

Train staff members properly. If they sort all the files in alphabetical or numerical order before they begin refiling, staff fatigue in the filing process is reduced. Once the files are in proper order, the medical assistant need only scan for the out-guides, and replace the files in their proper order. This eliminates movement in refiling A, and then going to Z, and so on.

Medical records management has progressed a long way from the invention of the four-drawer filing cabinet in the late 1800s. Physicians no longer have to bear the many aggravations of antiquated record keeping systems. With the age of computers, there will be a transition to more effective use of records, but these changes depend on well-organized systems.

●

Chapter 24

Collection Strategies

Financial arrangements with patients should be well thought out and documented in this competitive era. Credit and collections, if not handled carefully, can weaken the positive relationship with your patients and can lead to a large patient turnover in your practice. This area can cause great friction for you, your staff, and your patients. Time spent in implementation of effective credit systems in your practice will yield significant returns in your practice enhancement program.

Prudent fiscal decisions will have to be made, especially through inflationary and recessionary times, as patients' incomes and spending habits change. You will have to be prepared to strengthen or loosen your credit policies, depending on the requirements of patients and other considerations. In an underserved area, you should make your credit policy as stringent as possible. If there are more patients seeking your help than you can serve, it is to the benefit of your paying patients not to subsidize those who do not pay. Therefore, stringent credit and collection policies should be followed. However, as times change and patients' attitudes about credit change, you should also change along with them.

Credit cards have led to new types of financial arrangements. In the future, we will see a relaxing of policies calling for payment at the time of service, which will be replaced by a greater use of credit cards. Cash payments for services have decreased significantly as credit cards gain prominence.

It has been shown in business that the granting of credit will allow businesses to expand. However, credit arrangements should be controlled to ensure that bad debts are kept to a minimum.

Policy Suggestions

The following suggestions should help with your credit and collection policies:

Obtain Credit Information

Have patients fill out a comprehensive credit and collection form before granting them credit. The more information you can get about your patients, the more you will be able to use this information to find patients who have left town or who have been difficult to collect from. This comprehensive credit form will also allow you to begin building a data base on various patients in your practice and their credit histories. From this data base you will be able to make prudent decisions on practice collection policies.

Communicate Your Credit and Collection Policies

Credit and collection policies should be clearly communicated to your patients. This can be done by means of written materials, by telephone communication, or in person when the patient arrives. The key to a successful credit and collection system is how well your patients understand your procedures and how well your staff members implement those procedures.

When you have already informed your patients over the telephone what your fee is, they know before they arrive what they will be charged and they will be much more comfortable when presented with the bill. Also, if the fee is greater than they had anticipated, they will be able to ask and the difference can be explained to them.

Provide Private Space to Discuss the Bill

Your office should be designed to ensure a private place out of earshot of other patients, where your receptionist can discuss the bill with the patient. Many patients are reluctant to let your staff know about their financial situation in front of other patients who are waiting in the reception area. In addition, they are often more willing to pay at the time of service if it is done in a separate, private area.

Follow a Strict Collection Timetable

If patients can expect a bill at a regular time from your practice, they will know that your procedures are tight and will be more apt to comply. As in any business, you should follow a strict credit and collection timetable to stay on top of your cash flow, and follow through with dunning notices as required.

Send More Frequent Dunning Notices

A number of medical practices are starting to dun their patients more frequently than every 30 days. A number of studies have proven that if the patient does not send a check within two weeks after a first reminder, they are ready for another dunning notice. Therefore, in a 120-day period, you should consider sending four or five notices, and this will yield greater results than if you send only one.

Call Before Using a Collection Agency

Make sure you contact patients before sending them on to collection agencies. The personal telephone call from your office to the patient will yield you greater results in your collection efforts than any other single method. Many times doctors are caught up in the day-to-day routine and do not have enough time to call patients and follow up. Often a simple misunderstanding can be cleared up, or a problem explained, which will allow us to make the right decision about a collection issue.

Use a Calendar

Control all payment promises using the calendar. If a patient promises to pay within a certain time, this should be noted on a calendar and followed up on that particular date. If patients have failed to meet their promises, they should be notified, either through the mail or by telephone. By letting the patient know you are on top of things, you instill confidence in them and ensure that they pay.

Figure 24-1

Accounts Receivable Aging Summary

	For Month Of		For Month Of		For Month Of	
	No. Of Accounts	Amount	No. of Accounts	Amount	No. of Accounts	Amount
Direct billing						
To be billed (1 to 30 days)	___	___	___	___	___	___
Aged balances (31 to 60 days)	___	___	___	___	___	___
Overdue (61 to 90 days)	___	___	___	___	___	___
Past due (91 to 120 days)	___	___	___	___	___	___
Delinquent (over 121 days)	___	___	___	___	___	___
With collection agency	___	___	___	___	___	___
To be written off (less than $10)	___	___	___	___	___	___
Credit balances	___	___	___	___	___	___
Special accounts (reason _____)	___	___	___	___	___	___
Subtotal	___	___	___	___	___	___

Third-Party:

Medicaid

Medicare

Private insurance (pending)

Workmen's compensation

Other: _____

_____

_____

_____

_____

Subtotal

Grand Total

Send a Return Envelope with Your Bills

Many practices do not send return envelopes with their bills, which basically tells patients to pay that bill last. Since all other commercial companies send return envelopes, you should too. You will find this yields significant results in your collection efforts.

Set Up a List of Amounts Overdue

Figure 24-1 is an example of an accounts receivable aging list. You should consult this on a monthly basis to determine how far your accounts are sliding from month to month. Information should be recorded in terms of the number of claims as well as total dollars involved.

End the Doctor-Patient Relationship

Terminate the patient relationship if his or her account has been turned over to a collection agency. When a patient refuses to pay your bill and you have to go the lengths of turning that patient over to a collection agency, you should automatically terminate the patient relationship, using a registered letter with a return receipt requested. Patients who do not comply by making payment are not worthy of being in your practice. Remember, your paying patients are subsidizing those who do not pay, and you should not burden yourself with those patients who are constantly causing problems for you.

●

Chapter 25

Creative Facilities Planning Techniques That Maximize Patient Satisfaction

Have you ever stopped to wonder how you judge a favorite restaurant, boutique, or any business when you encounter it for the first time? Yes, reputation and quality of service are important, but (consciously or subconsciously) you judge a service establishment by many intangibles, such as the design and decor of the facility. This approach is also true of your patients. Many of them come to you because of your reputation and quality of your practice, but they judge you by the impressions they receive. A key element includes your decor and design of your facility.

The creative, pragmatic planning of your practice environment can significantly affect your practice growth. An attractive, well-organized practice environment helps to portray your concern for their comfort. Your facility can influence how relaxed patients feel, both physically and mentally. A well-planned space maximizes both your time and that of your staff members, thus making you more productive. Moreover, a well-planned facility will allow you and your staff to spend more quality time with your patients. A well-laid-out and carefully planned medical office environment focuses primarily on four areas, including (1) the reception room, which creates the initial impression; (2) the reception desk, where patients are greeted, and where they pay; (3) the examination room, where patients feel very vulnerable; and (4) miscellaneous areas, such as hallways, storage areas, and the like. The rest of this chapter contains specific suggestions for some of these areas.

Your First Impression—The Reception Area

Upon entering your vestibule, what is the patient's first impression of your practice? Next time you go into your office, use the front door rather than the back door and have a look around. Does it project a warm, welcoming feeling or is it shabby, dirty, and uninviting?

In place of a coat closet, I recommend pegs for coats, with a boot rack underneath. Amenities such as a mirror in the coat area or an umbrella stand nearby are appreciated by patients.

Consider the initial impression that the patient has of your receptionist. Is there an impressive and open feeling that encourages communication between the medical assistant and the patient? The same applies to your office. If your office projects a warm, caring, and calming atmosphere, it also facilitates the same open communication.

One problem in many doctors' offices is the proliferation of signs. In addition to your initial greeting, I generally recommend two key signs: a "No Smoking" sign and one that says "We appreciate payment at the time of service." More than two signs will never be read. If a notice is important enough to be put up, you should make sure it is professionally produced and framed, so that it fits with the image you are trying to project.

While the reception area should be in full view of the patients, the receptionist should be able to close off this area by sliding a glass partition for a confidential discussion with patients about either financial matters or medical issues. (Notice that I said *reception area*, not *waiting room*, since the latter term connotes a prolonged, uncomfortable wait; the term *reception room* gives the feeling that you will be received warmly, in a comfortable environment.)

Your reception room should be decorated in as high a quality of furniture, fixtures, and decor as will be accepted by your patient population. To decorate your reception area with expensive antiques and furnishings would not be appropriate if you have primarily a blue-collar, working-class practice. However, if you have an upper-middle-class practice, you would consider upgrading your reception area. As a rule of thumb, your reception area ought to be decorated a little better than the average living room of the patients in your practice.

Lighting

Lighting plays an important part in projecting a warm feeling. Replace all fluorescent lights in your reception area with track lighting or pot lighting in the ceiling. Lighting should be adequate for reading, but not harsh.

Reading Materials

Have built-in magazine display racks mounted to the wall, and eliminate all coffee tables and end tables, to create a more spacious feeling in the reception area. You can purchase special plastic covers to prevent magazines from becoming torn and dog-eared.

Children's Area

An important feature to consider in your reception area is a children's play section separated from the rest of the reception area. One doctor has a custom-built area for children to play in, with an enclosed fish tank that they can step up to and examine the fish. Many children can be occupied for a long period of time by looking at an attractive fish tank.

In family practice, psychiatry, and some other specialties, consider putting a one-way mirror from the interior offices to the children's play area so that the children may be observed at play.

Seating

Seating should consist primarily of individual armchairs or tandem seats with common arms. These should be comfortable and firm, and not so deep as to create difficulties when patients rise from the chair.

Carpeting

Wainscotting—bringing the carpet partially up the wall—is attractive and protects the walls. It also seems worth completely carpeting the walls in the children's play section.

Optional Patient Amenities

You might include a telephone that can be used by the patients in the reception area. However, I recommend a wall-mounted telephone, with no chairs around, so that patients will be discouraged from monopolizing the telephone for long periods of time.

A music system should be wired in with ceiling microphones, and it is a good idea to include the option of paging your patients if necessary. Although this is somewhat controversial, I recommend that the reception area have a television set, which can be used for viewing popular shows or for patient education. One ophthalmologist who specializes in cataract surgery has an oversized 6 × 6 foot screen and uses the television to play patient education videotapes on the subject of cataracts.

A water cooler or coffee machine in the reception area is an additional patient amenity. Patients also enjoy the presence of bulletin boards with community items, newspaper articles about your patients, and pieces about you and your staff. Many specialists in obstetrics and gynecology have bulletin boards in the reception area where patients can display pictures of their children.

The Heart of Your Practice Operations—The Business Office

Since the business office is so important in your practice operations, its design should ensure patient confidentiality and the provision of a high level of service within the facility.

As already mentioned, the reception area needs to be open, but provision must be made for private discussions about financial matters or confidential medical problems. The design of the business office, therefore, as well as its location, is of prime importance. It should be central to the patients, yet far enough away, or separated by a sliding glass partition so that discussions cannot be overheard by patients sitting in the reception area.

Generally, in service areas of hotels, airline check-in counters, grocery stores and the like, stand-up counters are utilized. In a medical practice, these establish patients and staff at an equal eye level, and improve communication between the two. I highly recommend the use of stand-up counters in your reception area.

Examination Rooms

Generally speaking, the examination rooms should be mirror images of each other—that is, except for expensive equipment costing over $250, each room should be similarly equipped. Try to lay out each so it is a model of efficiency. Wall mounts should be used for as many of the instruments (such as blood pressure cuffs) as possible.

Miscellaneous Amenities in the Examination Room

Some physicians, rather than placing white paper sheets over the examination table, use paper with designs such as colorful flowers.

Doors to examination rooms should be at an angle that does not permit a clear view into the room when the door is partially open. The patient should be shielded at all times.

Both indirect and fluorescent lighting should be used in the examination rooms. When you are talking with the patient you can have the indirect lighting on, while the fluorescent lighting is used while examining the patient. You can create two ambiences in the room.

A final amenity, which also adds to your efficiency, is to install a call button in the examination rooms. This will allow you to keep talking with the patient; if you need assistance, you can just press the call button.

Other Miscellaneous Amenities

A number of medical offices are now installing conference rooms off the reception area, to allow physicians to have meetings for purposes of patient education. These also serve as good lunch areas and physician conference rooms. One of your main objectives in designing your space, in addition to creating a warm and relaxes environment, is that it should be a model of efficiency. This does not imply a production line practice. By structuring the practice in such a way that patients can be moved from the reception room into the business area and clinical examination rooms in an efficient, effective manner so that your time and that of your staff is maximized, you will be developing an excellent model of service and patients will develop confidence in you and your practice as a cost-effective deliverer of health care.

The pursuit of creating an environment that reflects concern for the patient as well as efficiency for the doctor and staff is an ongoing challenge; however, in this competitive era, the atmosphere of your facility will differentiate your practice in a major way.

———————————————————————————●

Chapter 26

Financial Accounting Systems

Mary, my receptionist/bookkeeper, seemed to be one of the most loyal and devoted employees I ever had. She was always in the office long after everyone had left, worked weekends to catch up on book work, and even took work home with her. Everything went well for five years, until she suddenly became ill and we had to bring in a replacement.

During her absence, we found that the books wouldn't balance. When the accountants were brought in to train the new person, they discovered that large sums of money were missing. We estimate that more than $25,000 was embezzled over the past five years.

Embezzlement is just one critical area that needs to be examined in an overall evaluation of a practice's financial system. Most financial accounting problems result from inadequate accounting systems. By implementing a regular reporting system for the income and expenses of your medical practice, you can protect your practice from loss and anticipate potential problems.

Yours Is a Small Business

What can a good accounting system do for you? (1) A financially sound practice, which should result from such an accounting system, enables you to provide your patients with the amenities and level of service they require. (2) Certain financial systems can ensure your practice's future solvency. (3) Good accounting techniques help you evaluate your practice's financial health, enabling you to have a sound basis for decision-making.

Your Financial X-ray

Your regular income statement and balance sheet are the financial x-rays of your practice. They let you know how your practice has done during the period examined and give you a good measure of its financial health. Every one to three months, you should meet with your accountant or advisor to review your financial statements and examine any changes. You should analyze key expense categories, such as staff salaries and supplies, and compare them with those of previous periods. Many physicians could have avoided serious financial problems if they had instituted monthly reporting; they could have seen the problems early and been able to react quickly.

Figure 26-1 shows a form for a financial report; I recommend that you adopt some comparable report in your practice. A statement of this type can help you keep track of the changing financial situation on a month-to-month basis.

When examining your financial statements, pay attention to your gross fees generated and collections, as well as on your larger expenses such as salaries. A valuable analytical tool is an analysis of your current month's gross income and expenses. Compare them with those of the same month last year, paying special attention to any category with a variance.

Financial reports also limit potential loss in the practice. By listing projected budget and expenses, you will be constantly monitoring changes in the practice. Should the financial reports not reflect what you feel ought to have happened in a particular month, you can examine things more closely. In addition, good, tight financial systems should help your practice stay profitable.

Prevention of Embezzlement

The main reasons for the high rate of embezzlement in medical practices are high staff turnover, lack of financial controls, and the fact

Figure 26-1

Monthly Practice Financial Report

For month of _____

	This Month	%	Aver. Month Yr. to Date	%	Budget	%	Yr. to Date	%
Receipts:								
Practice								
Other								
Total receipts		100%		100%		100%		
Operating expenses:								
Staff salaries								
Fringe benefits								
Rent/utilities								
Bus insurance								
Medical supplies								
Office supplies								
Dues & subscriptions								
Telephone & answering service								
Auto & travel								
Library								
Fees—accounting, legal								
Loans								
Taxes								
Maintenance								
Miscellaneous								
Total practice expenses								
Practice revenue								

Misc. expense										
Prof. salaries										
Misc. salaries										
Fringe benefits (pension & profit sharing)										
Loans & interest										
Prof. education—meetings & seminars										
Enter. & promo.										
Misc. expenses										
Contributions										
Depreciation										
Total misc. expenses										
Net practice income										

that all financial matters are delegated to one person. I would make the following recommendations:

Bond All Staff

Fidelity bonding, preferably a blanket bond, is recommended for all staff members. Bonding is simply insurance that will reimburse you for the amount of the embezzlement. Bonding is also a deterrent, since the bonding company will always prosecute the alleged embezzler. It is a good precautionary tool to have implemented in every practice. Since all businesses that handle cash bond their staff, from local department stores to fast food outlets, there is no reason why you should not do the same.

Read and Understand the Checks You Sign.

You should be signing your checks twice a month, all at the same time. When you do this, instruct your staff to make sure that the invoice is with the check, and to scrutinize the invoice carefully, noting to whom the check is made out. You should always know whose checks you are signing. By the way, never leave blank, signed checks around the office.

Formalize Your Petty Cash Expenditures

Petty cash expenditures should be formalized; that is, each expenditure on petty cash should be substantiated with a receipt in a petty cash fund. I recommend buying petty cash books and a number of petty cash receipts from your local stationery supply.

Try to Break the Chain by Having Two People Work on the Financial Accounting

The best way to break the embezzlement chain is to have more than one person work on the accounting. Ideally, your accountant or spouse would handle the reconciliation of the bank book, and your medical assistant would handle the day-to-day transactions.

Conduct an Index Card Audit

An index card audit is a simple way of checking to see that all charges and receipts have been recorded for that day. Simply carry along with you a small index card in your pocket, and note the name of every patient you see and the charges that you had. Later, check that all charges have been entered into your daily accounting system.

Make Sure You Have a Check Protector Machine

A check protector machine, which costs about $100, safeguards you against mail fraud and forgery. It perforates your checks so that it is not easy to alter them—a good investment for total financial control.

Have a Professional Audit Conducted

A good use of your accountant's time is to have him or her complete a professional audit at least once every three years. This will give you the peace of mind that everything is in order in the practice. You will also get a number of suggestions for improving the internal controls in your practice.

Formalized financial controls and management are critical to the success of your practice. Make sure that your books balance daily, that you know your current cash position and your accounts receivable, and on a monthly basis that you know specifically how your practice is doing.

Review your financial situation at least on a quarterly basis with your advisors and be prepared to make fiscal changes quickly. As times are changing, you must be able to adapt financially.

Good financial systems are the lifeblood of any business, and this is especially true in a medical practice. Why? You know how hard you have to work to earn your money—make sure you keep it.

●

Chapter 27

The Computer: A Practical Tool for Enhancing Your Practice

An interesting romance between physicians and computers has been occurring since the mid-1970s. The lure of tremendous potential for office efficiency, productivity, and improved patient care coupled with a certain toy appeal and status has captured the imagination of physicians throughout North America. Computers have been touted as an instant cure for practice management ills. Many systems have been sold and integrated within physicians offices; however, a huge number of systems have become expensive dust collectors, have caused much frustration, and become excellent ways for doctor's children to do their homework or play games.

As we enter the competitive era and see large price reductions in computer hardware and software, you no longer need to struggle with the issue of whether or not you will be purchasing a computer. The main issue is when you are going to buy it, how you are going to buy it, and most importantly how you are going to make it work. A computer can be an effective tool in the development of a comprehensive practice enhancement program. Computers can be especially effective in managing your patient data base—that is, the analysis of patient demographic information and the use of this data base as part of your marketing program. If effectively integrated, computers can also assist you in collections, management reporting, cost control, and personnel management. With the integration of telecommunications with computerization, your telephone may also be part of your computer system.

Organized medicine is also getting actively involved in the standardization and direction of computer systems. The American Medical Association, in a joint venture with G.T.E. Corporation, has developed a comprehensive medical data base network that allows physicians to access the network and communicate with each other. The potential uses for such a network are enormous.

As we consider the new technology, it is important to understand what a computer can do for us and also what it cannot do. To avoid turning your purchase into a dust collector, you must clarify your specific objectives as to what you expect from it in your practice, understand the trade-offs, and finally decide how to implement it and make it work in your practice.

What Can a Computer Do For You

There are many misconceptions about what a computer can do for your practice. You should make a careful assessment of your reasons for purchasing a computer system. If all you need is an efficient manual procedure, make the change to that procedure before integrating your computer. This will allow you to see how smoothly you can function without the additional cost and expense-control of a computer system.

Will a Computer Reduce Staff?

Staff reduction might occur in a group practice, but in small practices manual procedures can accomplish about as much as can be done by computer if you are using efficient systems and procedures. A solo practitioner will find it difficult to get by with any less than two people. In every practice there is some "down time," and your staff might be doing many of the tasks that you might want a computer to do when you are not in the office. Computers might reduce some part-time expense if you are in an extremely busy practice.

Can Computers Reduce Your Management and Supervisory Responsibilities?

It has been my experience that good computer systems force you to effect strict systems and procedures in your practice, thus reducing your management and supervisory responsibilities. However, you will find yourself spending about the same amount of time in managing your practice, but you will be doing it with better information since your computer will be able to print more comprehensive records. You will have at your finger tips definitive data on patient demographic characteristics, financial activity, and practice costs. As a result of this information you will have more knowledge to make practical management judgments and decisions.

Can Computers Reduce Staff Involvement in Task Completion?

Computers are very good at performing repetitive tasks; however, other than filling out forms for insurance reimbursement, there are very few repetitive tasks in a medical office.

In my observation, many of the tasks in a doctor's office are completed by using shortcuts based on judgment. Because computers cannot apply judgment to the management of a medical office, some practices that have computers have found that the staff spends more time in practice management routines. The increased time results from the fact that the computer system requires certain steps to be completed before you can go on to the next step. A discipline is injected into the system, forcing your staff to complete each step of the task, steps that they may have skipped in the past. I feel that this is a benefit since your overall practice systems and procedures will be more complete as a result of the input.

Can the Computer Provide More Management Data and Other Useful Information?

Computers are good at storing a lot of data; as a result the reports coming out of a computer can be voluminous. Many practices receive 50-page computer reports that are produced monthly and read by no one. If you are getting the computer for more accurate management information, you want to be sure that the reports produced are simple and easy to understand and that you are actually going to use the information from the computer.

As a general rule, I feel that it should be possible to reduce every management report to one page. A report that is over one page in length is excessively complicated to read and understand, and it lacks a clarity in practice management direction. This is especially true for management reports. The exceptions, of course, are staff working reports, such as those dealing with collection call follow-up or appointment reminder calls. These reports are usually as long as they need to be to get the job done.

Can the Computer Reduce the Amount of Paper Work?

Another misconception is that the computer can reduce much of the work in the office. It has been my experience that a number of medical practices operate very inefficiently, especially in processing paperwork. With a little bit of thinking and time you will find that you can reduce many of your repetitive tasks simply by understanding the most efficient manual procedure. Many times all computers do is replace your antiquated manual system with a more efficient one, but a better manual system may be preferable.

Know What You Want Out of Your Computer

Your objectives for your computer should be clarified if you really want to use your machine for anything other than game playing, status, and toy appeal. Therefore, you should decide specifically what you want your computer to do before you purchase it.

Having said all this, I feel that the purchase of a computer for your practice is still a wise decision. My caution is that for a computer system to be truly effective in your practice, you want to delineate your objectives for computerization clearly and measure those objectives with the actual results you achieve once you get them into practice. After all, all that counts is that when you purchase it, it works and does the job you expected before that buying decision. You do not want a valuable tool to collect dust and add little or nothing to your practice.

Key Uses For Computer Equipment

The majority of computers purchased by medical practices are used mainly to do billing and accounts receivable control. This is the area that has been perceived by physicians and management experts to have the largest payoff. It is also the area with the most repetitive tasks that maximize the storage capability of a computer.

Other important uses for your computer include collecting patient demographic information, diagnoses, and procedures; this information can be evaluated in terms of practice costs and financial information to determine the most viable avenues for practice growth and expansion in the future. You will also be able to improve patient compliance by storing critical follow-up dates at your discretion.

Cost containment and financial control should also be a key objective of your computer system. All your practice financial records should be entered into the computer, and you should receive monthly management reports that list your volume and practice profitability. Reports should indicate changes in practice financial condition and patient growth.

Research is another area in which your computer should be useful. By storing information on diagnostic procedures and patient demographics, you will have easy access to data about specific trends in your practice. As a result the ability to publish papers or retrieve charts of patients with specific problems will be enhanced by integrating the computer in your practice.

A highly overlooked area in medical practices, especially in specialty practices, is the use of the computer for word processing. This is especially effective if you write many consultation letters. Computers can store standard paragraphs and information that are used routinely. In primary care, word processing is now being used in preparing patients' charts, with associated checklists and flow sheets.

Although computers can replace your appointment book, they cannot do the scheduling in your practice. Too much judgment and sophistication is required for the computer to schedule your patients effectively. As a result, great flexibility has to be built in to your appointment scheduling system if computerizing it is one of your goals.

Telecommunications should be a prime objective of computerization. The combined project of the American Medical Association and G.T.E. will allow you to dial into a medical data base with access to current information as well as a network to communicate with other specialists in any field on any particular problem. The program allows physicians to get close to computer-assisted diagnosis, and the data base has tremendous ramifications. Therefore when considering a particular computer system, its adaptability for telecommunications should be critical in the overall decision-making process.

The Trade-offs

It has been my experience that the cost of hardware and software is only a minuscule part of the cost of computer systems. The most expensive part of the computer purchase is learning time, conversion time, and your investment in the entering and use of data in the computer. If your time is worth $150 per hour and it takes you the 15 hours estimated by experts to learn any one piece of software in your practice, then the software package for which you paid $500 actually costs an additional $2,250 of your time. After you add your staff time in learning the package, and also the cost of conversion, you can see that your $500 purchase is well over $5,000 in terms of time spent in making it work.

Another trade-off is the servicing of the computer. Will the service be performed at your practice or will you have to carry the computer to the computer shop. When you have a computer problem it is rarely something simple. It might require three or four trips to the computer shop until the equipment is finally fixed. Therefore on-site service is desirable although it costs significantly more.

Another consideration is the continuing management responsibility of the system. When you purchase an integrated system where the hardware, software, training and support are all provided by one company, then the responsibility of that company is to make it work. Many times the purchaser buys hardware from one company, software from another, and support from a third. In such cases the purchaser often finds that the hardware service people point at the software people as the problem, and the reverse. And when all else fails, the cable that connects the computer to the printer can be blamed. The ideal computer for your practice would be the one where the vendor manufactured the machine, wrote the software, supported the software, supported the hardware, and assisted your staff with problems and training. In this case if something does not work, you know who is responsible.

The successful installation of a computer in a practice involves an integration of good hardware decisions, good software decisions, and most importantly support and service. I place more emphasis on the support and service than on the hardware.

Making it Work

The critical question is, who will make the computer work? When analyzing the low-cost versus the high-cost systems you often find that you basically get what you pay for. For example if you purchase a higher-priced business computer system costing about $10,000 to $15,000, the vendor takes the responsibility for training your staff and integrating the system into your practice. Generally, the higher the cost of the computer the more training and assistance you get.

You therefore have to assess how much time you want to spend with the system personally. If you want to practice medicine and not bother with it, count on paying a lot of money for support. You need to decide whether you are going to be the pivotal person in the implementation of the computer or whether your spouse or someone in your office has an interest in making it work. In my experience, if there is no one continually pushing the implementation of the computer in your practice then it will gather dust.

One alternative might be to hire a computer student at one of the local universities to help in the integration. Some consultants suggest that you find the program and then go out and find the machine the program works on. The cost of a computer installation goes far beyond the purchase of the hardware and software.

When purchasing a microcomputer from a computer store, the objective will be to get as close to the system provided by the high-end dealers with less of the headaches. However, the headaches can never really be eliminated because you basically get what you pay for in computers.

At a minimum, if you are not sure that computerization is for you, you should buy one of the inexpensive machines to bring into your household so that you can start to get familiar with computers and their capabilities.

Finally, whether or not you purchase a computer system, you can see that it has many benefits. It can greatly improve your ability to enhance your practice and improve your viability in the marketplace. The computer can be a positive practice enhancement tool; moreover it will increase the overall quality of delivery of services to your patients and improve your ability to compete in the marketplace.

You and Your Colleagues

Your medical practice involves a complex interrelationship of patients, staff, systems, and care. Ultimately, it is a reflection of your philosophy and attitude about treating patients and doing business. A successful practice is a successful business, and it has as its customers your patients and your referral sources. Are your philosophies regarding practice enhancement evident through techniques of handling the patient, effective personnel management, efficient systems and procedures, and methods of dealing with your colleagues? You are the captain of your ship; therefore, you are responsible for the course your practice takes.

If your practice thrives, it will be because you implemented decisions and strategies congruent with your personal philosophies of practice, in addition to the quality of patient care you have been providing. Your personal style is crucial in the overall impression your patient has of your practice. Chapter 28 discusses the elements of your personal style.

The way that you handle patients on the telephone also affects practice success, and Chapter 29 develops this important practice variable in detail. Not only must you understand your personal style and how your patients and your referral sources respond to it, but you must also be keenly aware of what in your practice determines its value.

To be efficient and be able to offer a high level of service it is important that you delegate to make good use of your time. Delegation allows you and your staff to extend more services to patients. Chapter 30 describes the different methods of effective delegation and shows how it can help your practice enhancement program. The ability to delegate must be developed as a part of your personal philosophy of a medical practice as a business and your personal philosophy of working with staff.

Your referrals are the life blood of your practice. Chapter 31 discusses the development of intraprofessional referrals. Only by seeing the process of generating referrals as an integral component to your practice enhancement program will you be able to influence practice growth.

Positioning your practice in the patient's or referral source's mind is a crucial marketing principle that will become more important as competition increases. Practice positioning is a marketing concept that shows you how to capture a spot in your patient's mind. Only by understanding your practice intimately will you be able to plan disposition. You have to visualize your practice's position in terms of the competitive marketplace and how your patients perceive you. Chapter 32 develops the idea of practice positioning and how it affects you and your colleagues.

As your practice grows, as you decide to open up a satellite facility, or if you are planning for future growth, you need to understand the implications of choosing a partner. Chapter 33 discusses methods for making an effective choice of another physician in a competitive era.

The ultimate responsibility for practice success and survival lies with its leader. You need to understand yourself, your practice as a business, and the ways that you can stimulate referrals. Chapter 34 has details about setting a value on the business that is your practice, and Chapter 35 develops the concept of practicing medicine as a business. In coming to terms with this concept, you will be addressing the delicate balance between running a business and providing the best possible personal medical attention you know your patients deserve.

Your practice reflects your philosophy, personal style, and aspirations. To survive in the competitive era, you will need to ensure that your practice as a whole truly reflects your philosophy.

———●

Chapter 28

Implications of Your Personal Style

Your personal style and image will affect your patients more than any other variable in your practice. Remember, a visit to the doctor's office is an important event in any patient's life. Patients will be paying close attention to everything you say and do. They will be looking for clues to evaluate your concern and compassion for them personally and they will be trying to assess your competence as a physician and your overall outlook on quality. Therefore, the encounter with your patients should be carefully orchestrated from beginning to end.

To understand your personal style, you need to understand yourself, how people perceive you, and the way that this fits within your practice enhancement program. Your attitudes about quality, cleanliness, service, and value should be clear in your mind especially as they relate to your patient's visit to your office.

The process begins with communicating your philosophy to your patients, and it must be followed through in every aspect of the patient visit. You should pay close attention to those areas where your personal style may differ from the way that your patients want you to act. For example, the fact that you maintain a sloppy desk has little or no bearing on the quality of medical services you provide. However, if the untidiness makes you appear disorganized in your patients' minds, it will naturally

225

project the feeling that the medical care they are receiving is also disorganized. Remember, patients can judge the neatness of your office, but are not trained to judge you medically.

Consider How Your Patients Would Like You To Appear and Act

Of course, there can be no set rules for how you should act with patients. Each practice differs in style and delivery, and a critical variable in practice success is your ability to let your own personality shine through. However, there are some ideas that you can incorporate into your personal style to improve your patients' perception of you and lead them to think of your practice as being totally competent.

Patients usually appreciate physicians who look and act like professionals. They appreciate being seen on time, because it indicates to them that you are well organized, and that you think their time is valuable too. In fact, they appreciate it when you make sure that the total delivery of care is executed efficiently and pleasantly. They like to know you really care, as shown by the way you talk to them and treat them, and by the fact that you really listen to their problems. To succeed in private practice in the future, you will need to adapt your personal style to make it as pleasing to patients as possible.

Ways to Achieve a Positive Image

The following material outlines some ideas to improve your image with your patients:

1. See patients on time to let them know that their time is valuable too. By consistently letting your patients wait, you are signaling to them that you do not care enough about them to value their time. Waiting to see the doctor is the most major complaint patients have about their medical care. The longer patients wait, the higher their anxiety levels become, and the less confidence they have in your practice.

2. Always have your patients fill out a comprehensive form, including both patient demographic data and some preliminary medical history, prior to their visit with you. This demonstrates your thoroughness, saves you and your staff time, and gains valuable medical insight into the patient. It also helps the patient pass the time in the reception area while waiting.

3. Encourage your patients to write out specific questions they would like to have answered during the visit prior to seeing you. This helps you zero in on their expectations to ensure they get what they came in to see you for. It also facilitates the communication process by forcing questions to be committed to paper.

4. Arrange to have new patients arrive 10 to 15 minutes early so that a medical assistant can give them an orientation to the practice. This projects a professional image to the new patient and demonstrates a high level of service. It also orients the patient to the systems and procedures in the practice; by showing them how to be good patients, one can minimize patient compliance problems in the future.

5. Send a personal letter of welcome to all new patients in the practice. One doctor has special cards printed up for all new patients who walk into the practice; this represents a pleasant introduction to the practice before the patient arrives.

Let Personal Image Be Sensitive to Patient Wants

Before entering the examination room to see the patient for the first time, you should know his or her name and the reason for the visit. If your assistant places the patient's chart on the outside of the examination room door you can quickly familiarize yourself with the person whom you will be treating. By using his or her name and referring to the chart from memory you appear more competent and project a warm, personal touch to your encounter. People like having their names spoken; it establishes a positive relationship right from the beginning.

Some doctors wonder whether they should use first or last names. My suggestion is that it is always safe to be conservative and to address your patients by their last names. Let them indicate if they prefer that you use their first names. A number of doctors make it a habit to allow their patients to call them by their first names. They feel that it does not detract from their professionalism and establishes rapport with patients.

When entering the examination room to see patients for the first time, how do you let them know you are glad to see them? Do you smile? Do you use their names? Do you shake hands? These are all demonstrations of your sincerity and caring. You should also establish eye contact early. Patients appreciate eye contact, and it projects the feeling that you are very attentive.

Before examining a patient, do you always make it a habit to wash your hands? Many doctors feel that this is an important aspect of the patient encounter; even if their hands are clean, they go through the ritual of washing them for the patient's benefit.

If it is a new patient who was referred by another doctor or patient, do you say something positive about that referral source? This encourages referrals and indicates that you appreciate them.

Say something to the patient that makes it clear you know him or her. One physician who keeps a social progress note on every patient can impress patients by remembering that they went on vacation several months before and asking them about it. The patients feel he has an excellent memory and is truly interested in them.

Pay close attention to your posture and dress. Dressing professionally enhances your total impression you make on your patient. Therefore, your grooming must be impeccable and your clothes ought to be pressed and tasteful. If you feel that you want to project a very professional image, consider wearing whites and do not forget your stethoscope. Some physicians, however, want to avoid a clinical stereotype; they always wear more casual clothing (never a white shirt). This, of course, is your own decision.

Finally, remember to ask your patients if there is anything else they need to know before they leave. This ensures that all their questions have been answered, and that you truly care about them and their anxieties.

The image projected from the carpet in your reception room to the paint in the examination room should truly reflect your philosophies of practice and personal style. The image projected by your facility and your staff is critical in building a busy, successful practice in these competitive times. Remember, you are the star, since patients are coming to see you. Consider seriously how you project yourself. Your practice should truly reflect the image you want patients to perceive. Your personal style and image are integral in a total practice enhancement program.

Chapter 29

Physician Telephone Technique

Communication with your patients is key to your success. We have discussed the value of image and a successful interpersonal relationship with your patients. Another area that needs to be addressed is managing the telephone. Since you make many calls to patients and referral services over the telephone, these must be efficiently and effectively handled. Successful telephone communications depends on the use of a system in which your staff assembles all the information necessary for each call in advance.

Schedule Your Call-backs

Studies have indicated that it is most efficient to schedule your call-backs. Moreover, by scheduling your call-backs you have freed the patient from the anxiety of wondering when you might call. When a patient telephones and asks to speak with you, the medical aide should offer assistance. If, after thorough screening, it is determined that the caller still needs to talk with you, the medical assistant should advise the patient that you will call back at a particular time. It is a good idea to give a general time such as "between 10 and 11 A.M." Thus the patient knows that you will not call before 10, and can make sure that the phone is not being used at the stated time.

Take Detailed Messages

The medical assistant should be instructed to take detailed messages so that you have enough information to make a judgment. If laboratory work or medical records need to be referred to, or if any information needs to be sought out, this should be done by your assistant before you return the call. When you do make the call, the complete message pad should be in front of you, along with the patient's records and all other necessary information. There should also be a short note containing feedback from the staff member who has put together all the information for you.

Have Your Staff Member Place the Call

It takes nearly half a minute in total from dialing to getting the correct person to the telephone. If you place the call yourself, you are not making good use of your time. Patients generally accept having a secretary make the initial contact before putting the doctor on the line. You may want to use your discretion with certain patients who might be offended by this practice. It has been my experience, however, that most people do not object to this procedure.

Always call back anyone whom your receptionist told you would call—even if this is a short telephone discussion to confirm an appointment, or give brief approval to an agreement. Remember, a number of salespeople who contact you could be potential referral sources, and your general attitude could be a factor.

Try to speak in lay terms, so that patients understand what you are telling them. All telephone discussions should be noted in the patients' charts. One doctor has her nurse make the notation in the chart as she talks to patients in the call-back period. It is important to ensure that your patients perceive you as being "available" to help them with their medical problems. Therefore, call them occasionally when they do not expect to hear from you, to ask how they are doing. For example, if you treat a child with an ear infection, have your nurse call the following day to check on the child. Most mothers greatly appreciate the extra support. In fact, this is something that most patients really appreciate, and such an approach is a good practice builder. If you are unable to handle these calls yourself, have your nurse call on your behalf.

Attention to Detail Regarding the Telephone

Your telephone communication is as critical as your face-to-face discussions with patients. Over a practice career, you spend countless hours with patients on the telephone, so use the time wisely. How you handle it will greatly affect the image of your practice and lead to increased patient satisfaction and practice efficiency.

—————————————————————————●

Chapter 30

Delegation of Responsibilities

It was 7 P.M., and Dr. Sam Jones was slumped over a pile of letters, reports, and telephone messages that needed his attention before he could leave for the day. As he took a bite of his lukewarm hamburger, he began to reflect on his day, and on his life in general. He sensed that his wife was fed up with his working till 11 P.M. every night. Staff members were becoming frustrated with his disorganization, and more importantly, his patients were beginning to bear the burden. He knew they were spending longer periods in the waiting room, for some had complained about it; he knew, too, by their conversation that some felt the doctor was not quite in tune with their particular case as he shuffled through thick medical records and paper work.

Not only was this doctor's practice frustrating for all, but it would be hard pressed to succeed bountifully in the increasingly competitive future. One reason for his difficulty is that he was unable to delegate responsibilities to subordinates. As more and more pressure is placed to contain costs and be efficient, more doctors will incorporate solid business principles into their practices. A central aspect in the practice enhancement program is delegation, which involves transferring lower-level tasks to well-trained assistants.

In the past, doctors have not delegated responsibilities because they felt that only they could perform certain jobs. However, with community colleges and universities training more paraprofessionals in medical office tasks, there are many talented and trained people to whom a wide range of tasks can be delegated, from simple copy typing to giving injections and handling minor treatments. This not only boosts the doctor's productivity, it also provides an opportunity for him to improve professional, financial, and personal objectives.

The Importance of Delegation

Delegation has many benefits. You will have more time and attention to devote to giving a high quality of patient care. You will free yourself to perform those tasks for which you were trained—namely, diagnosing and treating patients' illnesses and motivating them to care for themselves; at the same time you will be able to grow professionally. By constantly operating at your most effective level, you will be freeing yourself from worrisome details. Remember, if you had wanted to be a nurse, bookkeeper, or typist, you would not have spent all these years training to become a doctor.

When you delegate, you are not weighed down by details that can be handled by someone else. You are then better able to view your entire operation more clearly, and you have time to think about such important decisions as quality control, cost effectiveness, and overall patient satisfaction with the practice.

If you show your staff that you have confidence in their abilities you can promote initiative and enthusiasm—attributes that greatly enhance staff productivity. Appropriate delegation gives your staff an opportunity to work at their capability level. This gives your patients better value from your time because you can concentrate on higher level tasks. More time is available to give patients a more thorough examination. There is no way that you can spend a half hour with each patient doing a thorough history. However, if the history is delegated to a conscientious, well-trained aide, you will have the information you need and use your time efficiently.

Effective delegation can help you increase your output. You can see more patients, which makes you more efficient and also controls costs in your practice. Efficient delegation can help you finish on time and be home with your family earlier.

Practical Aspects of Delegation

You can delegate tasks to any staff member who is bright and willing enough to accept added responsibility. However, you should be sure that each person to whom you delegate has excellent training. Your staff should be thoroughly cognizant of documented systems and procedures for screening telephone calls, giving injections, and other medical tasks. Remember, you are responsible for what goes on in your own office, whether you have a direct hand in it or not.

Planning for Delegation

Sit down with pencil and paper and, as quickly as you can, write down as many tasks as you can think of that you perform on any sort of a regular basis. Show this list to your spouse or close colleague(s) to see whether there is anything that can be added. Check your local state laws governing what can be delegated. (For example, some injections must be given by a doctor.)

Figure 30-1. Sample form for activity/resource person delegation.

Activity	Person	Person	Person	Person
1.				
2.				
3.				
4.				
5.				
6.				
7.				
8.				
9.				
10.				

On another sheet of paper, list as many resource people as you know who have the potential for assisting you with some of the regular tasks you perform. Beside each person's name, list his or her hourly pay. This will add focus to your decision regarding who will do what. Use a form such as the activity/resource person delegation sheet shown in Figure 30-1. Write the names of your resource persons across the top and write the activities you want to delegate down the left hand column. Next, match a person to the task. If you do not have enough resource people available, you might have to consider hiring more staff.

Describe the Tasks

Before you delegate the activity to the appropriate person, you should write a description of the task and the way it should be completed. This

Figure **30-2.** Sample of a delegated activity sheet.

To: _____

From: _____

Date: _____

Due date (complete): _____

Subject: _____

Required end results: _____

Standard of performance: _____

Activity checklist: _____

Guidelines: _____

Resources: _____

Interim review (date or stage   Time framework: _____
          of completion):

          _____

can be detailed in the activity checklist area on Figure 30-2. In this way, your assistant will know the sequence in which you wish the task to be performed. Also, note whether there is a date due on a special project and specify any guidelines or expected standard of performance. These details leave little room for misunderstanding, and you have the assurance that the task will be performed to a high standard. Later this activity list can become part of your medical office manual.

Taking the Positive Approach

If possible, create a positive atmosphere, since people tend to tune out negatives. Before you begin, state what you are going to delegate and find out precisely what the learner knows about the job already. Try to make the learner see the interesting aspects of the job; for example, if you are delegating a certain filing task, rather than calling the position *file clerk,* why not designate the job as *records manager* and make the person responsible for all aspects of paper flow and records management in the office. In this way, the previous mundane job becomes one of some importance.

Whenever possible, do the instruction in the area where the job is going to be done and place the learner where he or she will be working. For instance, if you are delegating weighing the patient or taking his or her blood pressure, do the instruction in the examination rooms where the procedures are performed.

Focus on the Goals

When describing what you are delegating, begin with the desired end results (see Figure 30-2), which will give the learner the sense of where you are headed. If you are delegating the task of taking preliminary patient histories, for example, get out a completed form and show the end product first. Then start with the simple things next and move on to complicated details. If you start with the complex details, many staff members will tend to tune out the rest of the instruction.

Demonstrate the Technique

Whenever possible, demonstrate the job yourself and go over the activity checklist or job description, underscoring the important points; discuss only one point at a time. Instruct the learner patiently and do not try to force him or her to master several details at once. In the case of preliminary patient work-ups, have the learner watch you with a few patients.

After you have explained the task in detail, have the learner do it while you watch. That person should show you what he or she is doing, and discuss the key points while performing the task. Correct any errors in the process, over and over, until you feel he or she is comfortable with the activity.

Set Up Procedures for Handling Questions and Reviewing Performance

Make sure that when a problem or question arises your staff reports it immediately. This is an excellent training method, and additionally it will make you feel more comfortable about delegating since you will feel you are in control. Also, it keeps you covered legally. I would emphasize to the staff that they be extremely cautious in this area, especially with the new public consciousness of malpractice.

Interim review dates should be established to check that each task is being performed in accordance with your desired standards. I would suggest that reviews, which can be written on a sheet, be frequent in the first few days or weeks after the activity has been delegated.

Since you will probably be delegating many tasks to a number of resource persons simultaneously, an activity control sheet (Figure 30-3) has been designed to assist you.

The most important aspect in the delegating process is that you control or monitor all delegated tasks. This ensures that quality of care and service to your patients remains at a high level. The implementation of effective delegation in your office will require some time spent in rethinking, reorganizing, and retraining. However, once the system is in place, you and your staff members will be better able to work at your most efficient levels most of the time. The advantages of this increased efficiency will lead to greater productivity for you and your staff and to more comprehensive care for your patients.

●

Chapter 31

Working with Referral Sources

Managing your referral sources for practice growth is a critical variable to practice success. Physicians in specialty practice rely more on referrals from other professionals rather than on direct patient referrals. However, it is still patient satisfaction with your service that will directly affect your practice growth.

It has only been during the past few years that direct physician referrals have accounted for the major part of patient activity. After the fifth year of a practice, patient referrals tend to be more important as a factor in practice growth. For example, a patient who had a hernia operation performed by you as a result of a referral from a family practitioner will tell other patients how good a doctor you are. Therefore, when it comes time for surgery, other patients may request to have you as their surgeon. Or, more important, if the referring physician gives the patient a choice of surgeons, he or she is apt to decide on you based on favorable comments from other patients. In addition, patients who are satisfied with your service will go back and tell the referring physicians about the level of care they received. Thus, the referring physicians' decisions will be reinforced by positive recommendations from their patients.

To develop an effective referral generating program, it is critical to understand who your referral sources are, why they are referring to you, and how you can improve your service to them. From a marketing point of view, one could say that the referring professional is also the specialists' consumer. Therefore, your practice must be geared to meet their needs as well as the needs of their patients. Do you know for example, whether your referral sources would like in-depth consultation letters or short letters with key findings only? My surveys of primary care physicians show that about 50 percent would like in-depth letters, while the other 50 percent prefer short letters because they are easier to read. Have you surveyed your referral sources to determine what type of letter they would like to receive from you, or are you just cranking out the usual standard letters? You should also ask referring physicians whether they would prefer a personal telephone call about the patient's case rather than a letter. Make a note of the preference.

As discussed in the first section of this book, do you monitor your referral sources on an ongoing basis? Only by knowing what the level of activity from referral sources is can you begin to determine trends and make changes in your service.

You should have an active program to express appreciation for a referral. A special letter should be sent to a physician thanking him or her for the referral, apart from the actual consultation report. One doctor calls every new referral source personally and thanks him or her for the patient who was sent to him. Another has a special Christmas party every year at the best club in town, inviting all his referring physicians as a thank you gesture. When you are at the hospital or in a social situation, you should go out of your way to express personal thanks for support and referrals; this is a useful way to increase your referrals.

The major factor in building referrals is your provision of the service expected by the referring physician. The speed with which you report back to him or her about the patient's problems is an important component in determining that level of service. One radiologist has a 24-hour turn around time for all reports; to accomplish this, he has a staff member who delivers all reports by car at the end of each day for the previous day's work. That is service!

Although you may not be aware of it, one factor that greatly influences professional referrals is friendliness with colleagues. This means you have to budget an entertainment fund into your practice enhancement financial plan. It might mean one or two annual parties, taking out some of your key referral sources for dinner, or just general socialization. It is also important to remember anniversaries, births, and birthdays with a personal note or card. If there is a new grandchild in the family, be sure to send a personal gift. It is the small touches that really make a difference in developing your referral sources. If you can send patients to your referral sources in return—even only one or two patients when they have sent you 10—it is a step in the right direction.

Always do your best to work in any patients of your referring physicians as soon as possible. Remember, availability is one of the biggest practice builders; even though your practice may be well established, your biggest referral sources may change their patterns if they cannot get their patients in to see you early enough.

Where possible, you should try to involve the referring physician in the process of caring for the patient. A number of primary care doctors have expressed the feeling that they will not refer patients to a specialist to whom they lose control. They want to be involved in the process and consulted each step of the way regarding all later referrals. Therefore, you should never send a referred patient to another physician without touching base with the initial referral source.

Other ways of increasing your visibility to build referrals include teaching at the hospital, medical school, or medical society, attending meetings on areas of your expertise, and participating in general community and political activities. Publishing scientific papers and writing articles also increase your visibility in the practice and remind your referring doctors that you are competent and qualified.

As part of developing a referral management program you should set up a calendar of events for the development of your referral base. As a goal, you should have one activity set aside per month, over a 12-month period. These could include Christmas parties, Thanksgiving cards, personal contacts, lunches, and educational meetings (which you might sponsor). Use your creativity as you develop your program.

In the past, physicians have not paid enough attention to the development of referrals in the practice. By focusing on a program, and understanding that professional referrals can be stimulated for growth, you will find you are in better control of your practice's future.

Chapter 32

Practice Positioning: Capturing a Spot in Your Patients' Minds

The marketing concept of positioning has an important place in a long-range practice enhancement program. Wellness clinics, executive health clinics, and prevention clinics all illustrate the positioning concept.

An executive health clinic can be used as an example of a positioning strategy. An internist in Chicago determined that a large portion of his practice consisted of busy executives, and these were the patients that he found most satisfying. He was attracting a number of geriatric patients as well as other types of patients. By renaming his practice the *Executive Health Clinic,* he positioned his internal medicine practice as one that specialized in the health care issues of executives. When geriatric patients who are not executives seek an internist, they would typically not call the Executive Health Clinic for services. As you can see, positioning your practice targets your growth in those areas you deem desirable. When executives are looking for a physician and see the name Executive Health Clinic, they would be more likely to call that clinic because they would feel that it will meet their specialized needs.

In positioning the practice as an executive health clinic, the internist began to develop specific health programs for executives, including such services as stress reduction and hypertension programs. He also purchased new equipment to provide more comprehensive services to the specialized group that was prepared to pay more. This is a good example of a targeted approach to positioning your practice.

Another positioning concept can be seen in the approach used by an obstetric and gynecologic group or a family practice group that provides comprehensive services to women. If a family practice group names itself the *Women's Health Center*, it will attract mainly women into the practice because of positioning, even though the physicians are trained family practitioners who are able to deliver care to all families. As a result, the programs offered and delivery of services will be tailored for women and be potentially more comprehensive. Women's health centers have been a very successful positioning concept that will play a prominent role in the medical marketplace in the future.

Other types of positioning concepts have already been established by traditional medicine. Family practice is a medical specialty that is well positioned; it appeals to people who are family oriented and who would like one physician to handle the whole family. The patient also has the choice of having an obstetrician/gynecologist for the women in the family, an internist for the men, and a pediatrician for the children.

Other specific positioning concepts include the nutritional clinic, the prevention clinic for those people who are interested in preventive medicine, the industrial medicine clinic, a children's clinic, and various other subspecialties. There are also some new positioning concepts such as pain centers, obesity clinics, and so on. A number of these undoubtedly will be fads, but over time we will find that certain concepts will proliferate and capture specific segments of the medical care marketplace.

A final concept involves practices positioned with respect to price policies. One example is the low-price, no-frills clinic. A segment of patients will respond to this approach, especially those who feel that medical care is too expensive. The core service will be the same but augmented service will not be enhanced so that the price can be kept low.

Private Practice Positioning

The no-frills approach, however, is laden with financial and service risks. The overall success of private practice depends on providing a personalized service. As you know, personalized service and attention can cost more but it is the overall quality you are striving for.

One positioning strategy for private practice might be to position the practice as a slightly higher cost, but highly specialized, service. Patients may be paying a little more on a fee-for-service basis; however, they will be receiving more augmented service for their health care dollar. There will always be a need for a quality service in the health system, and the higher priced, higher quality concept is one that is well favored and well understood by consumers in general.

As positioning begins to play a larger role in health care, you will need to determine specifically how your practice is being positioned among all the alternatives that patients have to choose from in your community. You will be making trade-offs based on what the competition is doing in your area. Let me leave you with this thought, which applies most appropriately to the whole concept: Position is everything in life— what is yours?

●

Chapter 33

Choosing a Partner

"I cannot handle all the patient demand," Dr. John Gordon, a busy San Francisco internist told his medical assistant at 7:45 P.M. on Tuesday evening. It was another in a long string of late office closings. It seemed there were not enough hours in the day to meet his patients' demands for his time and services. He had not taken a vacation in some time, and he was worried about patient service declining.

Just two years ago, Dr. Gordon had changed his location and hired a laid-off airline stewardess to be his medical assistant in the front office; he worked extremely hard at satisfying his patients needs. As a result patient demand for his services was strong, but in order to maintain a high level of service, he would have to extend his hours, and he really did not want to do that.

Dr. Gordon is a typical example of many physicians who started using practice enhancement techniques several years ago and are now reaping benefits in practice growth. With competition invading medicine rapidly, many physicians are beginning to extend their services and become more patient centered. One strategy to compete with the extended-hour facilities for example, is to share your office. Some practices are open 12 hours per day six days a week; this is accomplished by two doctors with two separate staffs sharing the office and hours.

As competition intensifies, more and more physicians will be associating, or taking on partners. This chapter delves into the implications of choosing a physician to be your partner. (It is important to define the difference between an associate and a partner: if you engage an associate, the relationship between you is that of employer and employee; on the other hand, a partnership entails a formal agreement to share in the ownership of the practice.)

Should You Bring in a Partner?

Let me use Dr. Gordon as an example to illustrate some key considerations. Often bringing in a partner or associate is the right solution to ease time pressures on a physician, but before Dr. Gordon can make this decision, a number of issues need to be considered.

Does a Need For Another Doctor Really Exist?

Analyze how far ahead a patient has to wait to see you for both acute and nonurgent problems. If patients regularly must schedule these appointments far in advance, patient demands on your time are regularly exceeding your availability, thus making the need for an associate or partner more plausible.

If you have stopped taking new patients, consider keeping track of patients who call your office asking for an appointment and are turned away. This will give you a good idea of how long it might take to build up the practice of a potential partner or associate. Are there any services your practice could give your patients that you are not currently delivering because of preference? Could or would a new partner perform these services?

Would an associate make house calls or perhaps deliver babies? Your practice may have grown because of your house call service; you want to ensure that any new person you bring on shares the same attitude regarding house calls.

Finally, analyze how much of your time you are allocating to each type of patient problem. If it appears to be declining below a level you are comfortable with, this would signal further pressures on your time and present mode of practice.

Do You Have The Partnership Personality?

Many physicians practice extremely well in solo practice; however, they do not share decision and policy making very well. If you have been used to doing things one way for 20 years, would you be willing to change if new ideas were suggested from an associate or partner? Your willingness to share control and responsibility for staff and practice direction is essential for the partnership to succeed. It is far better to find out before you enter into any arrangement that you do not have the disposition for it. It can save you a great deal of frustration.

Analyze The Financial Implications.

Typically, when a new doctor joins a practice, the greater patient load necessitates more staff, equipment, and facilities. Determine the cost of any new equipment that would have to be bought, and decide whether you would need new facilities. It is a fallacy that two physicians can practice for the same price as one. Some expenses can be saved— you can share high-cost equipment and save rent on some common areas, if you can work your hours out satisfactorily to maximize the use of the facility. In the long run, however, the extra doctor will increase expenses. If you still believe you should take on an associate, you can move on to the next step in your planning.

Analyze and Reorganize Your Office Systems and Procedures

Perhaps you have always wanted to replace those antiquated filing or accounting systems. Now is the time to do so. With an extra physician around, your existing office systems will be under strain. Anything you can do now to avert future problems will be a help. Sometimes, by analyzing your office systems and staff delegation policies, you can come up with some useful data.

In the example of Dr. John Gordon, after an analysis, he decided to hire a full-time registered nurse. By delegating some of the minor procedures to her, he was able to ease patients' demands on his time. Often physicians take on tasks that do not merit their specialized training. In some cases, the solution may be to ease the pressure through the addition of more staff.

If you decide to take on an associate, make as many positive changes as possible before the new doctor arrives. In this way, you will greatly assist the transition of your new colleague into your practice.

Recruiting the Ideal Associate

You should let as many people as possible know you are looking for a partner or associate. Your best sources are personal contacts. Discuss your needs with any medical schools in a 200-mile radius. Your best candidates will come from towns or schools within this area. You can also call the chiefs of the various residencies of your specialty within the same area; a follow-up letter should be sent after the initial personal telephone call. Both your colleagues at the hospitals and coverage group should be informed that you are looking for an associate. Also place classified advertisements in all the key medical journals. Typically, when someone is looking for a practice opportunity, he or she reads these pages quite closely. Consider spreading the word through medical supply salespeople, who are often in contact with final year residents. Detailpersons also know of physicians who might be interested in your situation.

It will take you about a year to find the ideal candidate. Starting your search in March and April is too late if you hope to find a good quality candidate in the final year of the residency program.

You should delegate the responsibility for recruiting a partner or associate to one person. Obviously, if you are in a solo situation, the responsibility will be yours. In a partnership or group, one person should manage the total process. This gives continuity over the hiring process.

It is important to assemble an information package that describes and promotes the positive aspects of your practice and your area. This might include a one-page description of your practice, including your philosophies and benefits, such as location, quality of facilities, and the staff. Any candidate would also be interested in information about the city or surrounding area. Most cities have industrial commissions that keep attractive brochures and statistics to attract business; officials at city hall may also have such material. These brochures are normally available to citizens of the community, and you can get them on request. This material is a useful addition to the package you will be sending to a potential recruit, and the professional advertising is already done for you.

As much screening of candidates should be done by telephone as possible. Time spent in the initial screening of physicians will save you many hours in the future. The initial telephone interview should be 10 or 15 minutes long, to see whether the candidate fits your criteria. These should be in line with the goals you set out for acquiring a new associate. If the candidate is farther than 500 miles away, consider doing the major part of the interview over the telephone until you are fairly sure this candidate will meet your needs. Before you commit yourself to bringing the candidate to your area for an interview, check his or her references.

You should already have received a curriculum vitae with references. Make some telephone calls to people at the medical school who may have known the candidate, as well as to personal friends in the particular town the candidate is from. Get as much information as possible before the candidate arrives.

Should you pay the candidate's expenses for coming to see you? Here are a few guidelines. When most businesses hire high-level executives who will earn $50,000 or more, they pay for both the executive and the spouse to make the trip. Since you are considering a life-time partnership, it is important to meet the spouse and ensure that he or she would be happy in the location. (It is very important that the spouse be encouraged to come along for the interview. In many cases, the doctor may be happy with the professional aspects of the location, but the spouse will not be sold on the location; in such cases the physician will usually not move.) You should at least pay for one-half of the traveling expenses of the physician and spouse. Some practitioners pay for the spouse's trip and the physician pays his or her own way.

A plan should be made for every minute of the potential recruit's and spouse's time while they are in your city. Remember that the process is a two-way street—you are trying to find out if the candidate will fit into your practice, and at the same time you are trying to sell the candidate on the opportunity that you have to offer. Therefore, a plan for the visit is critical. The candidate and spouse should spend at least a full day and an evening visiting the location and practice.

Consider scheduling a few office hours in the morning or afternoon so that the candidate can get a feel of flow within the office. You may consider involving the candidate with some of your patients, to see how he or she reacts. Make sure you take the candidate to your regular hospital and other key areas of medical interest. It is important to point out to the potential candidate all the positive professional aspects of the community. For example, if there is a medical school nearby, visit it.

Plan to involve the spouse in at least 50 percent of the professional activities. The rest of the time should be spent with someone who can show the spouse the best things about the community, such as schools, recreation facilities, and the like.

If at all possible, try to get the candidate to spend at least two days in your town. In most situations, the first day will be taken getting acquainted with the community, and the second in considering the opportunity. If you have decided on a particular candidate, try to get some feeling for his or her wishes during the visit. Allow the candidate a seven- to ten-day "cooling off" period, in order to reflect on what has transpired. If the candidate and spouse feel they have analyzed the advantages and disadvantages privately and at length, they will be more content with their decision and much less likely to be disenchanted later about any problems that may arise than they would if too hasty a decision were made.

Evaluating the Candidate

Even if you are looking for an associate, view the process in the perspective of hiring a future partner. Most good associates will end up as partners, and you are being short-sighted if you look only for an associate.

Experience has proven that physicians who have had similar training, who have gone to the same medical schools and perhaps to the same residency programs together, stay together the longest and make the best partners. This is mainly due to the fact that many of one's goals are formulated while going through medical school and residency. Try to determine the goals of your future partner and see if they are congruent with yours. One way to get at this information is to ask open-ended questions, such as:

1. What do you want out of life?
2. What is your philosophy of practice?
3. How do you see yourself 10 years from now?
4. Describe what you would consider to be the ideal practice.

Money Comes Last

Discuss the monetary aspects of the proposal last. Try to understand the candidate's perspective on money, since finances are probably the most frequently cited reason for partnership breakdown. One way to find out what the candidate thinks about money is to ask how he or she might feel about splitting income equally after expenses. Even if you are a strong believer in productivity in a medical practice, the answer to this question will give you many insights into the potential partner's attitude about money.

If the candidate's knowledge of remuneration formulas is limited and he or she states that an equal split would be fine, give him or her a better understanding of what might happen. For example, how would he or she feel if one of the partners spends a lot of time teaching at a local university while the other was carrying much of the practice load?

Similar life styles are very important to the success of the partnership. Look at such things as similarities in family background and ethnic origin;

if you are a nonsmoker the ideal candidate would most probably be a nonsmoker also. Remember too, that most successful relationships are built on mutual trust.

Spelling It Out

It is very important to spell out in detail the basis of an offer in an informal letter to the candidate. Get your lawyer to review the offer. This letter should include all the considerations that would be needed for the candidate to make a decision. These points would include the following:

1. A two- to four-week time limit should be placed on the acceptance offer.
2. A probationary period should be spelled out—probably three to six months—during which either party may decide to terminate the relationship without penalties.
3. Be very specific about the remuneration and other benefits. If there is a base salary, state the base. If there is a bonus, be very specific about how the bonus is calculated.
4. If there are increases in salary, base, or bonus, state how and when these are determined.
5. Vacation leave, sick leave, education leave must all be covered in the letter.
6. With education leave, decide how many days off you will grant, whether or not you are going to pay, and if so, how much you will pay for continuing medical education.
7. The letter is also a good place to specify exactly how an associate can buy into the partnership.
8. Try to establish a value for "good will" of the practice. Good will involves all those intangible things that have gone into building the patient flow into the practice. Get a professional advisor to evaluate good will, and try to come up with a number of buy-in approaches at the outset. This will eliminate some areas of disagreement in the future, when discussing the purchase of the practice.
9. Some practices show a very detailed calculation on what the practitioner's take-home pay will be after taxes, unemployment insurance, and so forth.

10. Be very specific on improvements that will be made to the practitioner's office space and put a budget on redecoration and new equipment.
11. Other considerations may be membership dues, journal subscriptions, and any other incidental expenses that may be covered in the practice.
12. Finally, if the new doctor is to be on call for a large proportion of nights or weekends (in the first few years), it is important to discuss this in the initial letter. It is also very important to define precisely what the potential candidate is going to be receiving in the future. This forms the basis of a very solid, long-lasting personal relationship with the candidate. Only by spelling out what you expect of the new person or what will be granted in the beginning, will a successful relationship evolve into the future.

This letter can be used as a basis for the future relationship, or, if desired, a more formal contract may be drawn up by your attorney.

During these competitive times, when services are being extended, and patient demand begins to grow in your practice, you want to be able to meet patient demands and keep your service at a high level. In some situations, adding another doctor can ease some of the pressure, as well as bring additional rewards, such as regular professional interaction in difficult cases. However, make sure that you carefully assess the demand for services and that there is actually a need for another physician.

If you are contemplating this move, you should be ready to make some sacrifices and invest the necessary time in the recruiting and practice preparation phase. What transpires in the initial three months of the relationship will have a lasting effect in the long-term partnership.

●

Chapter 34

Setting a Value on Your Practice

In a competitive era, patients become a scarce resource. For this reason, we will be seeing more physicians purchasing practices rather than building them. There are many benefits to purchasing a practice, but the largest benefit is the fact that you are buying a patient base that you do not have to build; this also gives you a competitive advantage. It is important when purchasing a practice to determine its correct value. The process of setting a value on a practice is also important if you are considering selling your practice—it may be worth more than you think.

Taking a financial x-ray of your practice is precisely what you do when you try to determine its value. By following the worksheets provided in this section, you will be able to set a value on your practice.

Valuing Tangible Assets

Tangible assets are easiest to value (Figure 34-1). These are "hard assets" on which a value can be placed by a professional appraiser; the value can also be determined by some good analysis and sound judgment on your own part.

Tangibles can be valued at (1) their original cost, or the cost you

253

Figure **34-1**

Practice Valuation Work Sheet—Tangible Assets

1. **Equipment and Furnishings** _____
   a   Business office equipment and furniture _____
   b   Reception room furniture _____
   c   Examination room furniture _____
   d   Specialized medical equipment and instruments _____
   e   Art objects and collectibles _____
   f   Miscellaneous _____
   g   _____ _____
   h   _____ _____
2. **Supplies** _____
   a   Medical supplies _____
   b   Business supplies _____
   c   _____ _____
   d   _____ _____
   e   _____ _____
3. **Leases** _____
   a   Leased equipment value _____
   b   Favorable space rental terms _____
   c   _____ _____
   d   _____ _____

---

4. **Leashold Improvements** _____
   a   Decorating _____
   b   Carpeting _____
   c   Fixtures _____
   d   Plumbing _____
   e   _____ _____
   f   _____ _____
5. **Accounts receivable** _____
6. **Real estate value** _____
7. **Medical records** _____
8. **Cash and equivalents** _____
   a   Checking account _____

b	Petty cash	_____
c	Prepaid subscriptions	_____
d	Stamp and postage meters	_____
e	Prepaid expenses	_____
f	_____	_____
g	_____	_____

Total tangible assets   _____

Practice value

(Tangible assets + intangible assets − liabilities) =   _____

paid for them; (2) the replacement cost, or what it would take for you to purchase that item; or (3) the depreciated cost, otherwise known as the book value. Often the depreciated or book value does not reflect the actual value of the asset.

Equipment and Furnishings

As a rule of thumb, equipment and furnishings up to two years old are valued at 70 to 80 percent of their original cost. Older items will usually fetch 25 percent of their original cost. As a cross check, go to used furniture showrooms and see how much equipment similar to yours sells for. Office equipment usually depreciates faster than medical equipment; therefore, expect to get less for it.

Price each item separately. Go through each area of your office making sure everything is counted and valued. There is a chance you could have art objects and collectibles. Some medical books can also be worth a great deal. In addition, values depend on personal taste; your furniture might be in excellent condition, but if it is gaudy lime green and pink it might be worth very little.

Supplies

Since most practices have about three months' worth of supplies on hand, an easy way to value them is to look at last year's total expenditure for medical and business supplies and divide it by four. Deduct 20 percent from the result and you will have an approximate value. It is usually a waste of time getting an actual cost of the supplies; except in allergy practices, they rarely have much value.

Leases

Leases, of either equipment or office space, are often overlooked in practice valuation. Typically, rented or leased equipment is paid off over a three- to five-year period. At the end of the lease, the purchaser can buy it at nominal cost. For example, in another two months, you may be able to purchase for $1 a typewriter that has been leased over five years. If the machine is worth $500, consider that sum in the valuation.

The lease on office space might be worth more than you would think. Suppose, for instance, you have a 1,000-square-foot office leased for an agreed rate of $10 per square foot. Today, the rate is perhaps $12.50 a square foot. Assuming that the space can be sublet and there are three years left on the lease, the value of that lease is 1,000 square feet × price per square foot per year × 3 years, or $7,500 in reduced rental payments over the three-year period.

Leasehold Improvements

Improvement to space, including painting and decorating, carpeting, plumbing, lead walls, and the like, can be included in the value. Typically, these leasehold improvements are amortized over a seven- to ten-year period by the landlord. Generally speaking, assume that the leasehold improvements are worth one-third of the original cost of the improvements, if they are more than three years old; allow one-half the original cost if they are less than two years old.

Discount any specialized leasehold improvements, such as special laboratory facilities that another tenant may not be able to use. Remember, improvements become the property of the landlord unless they are removable. You are actually paying for the use of the leasehold improvements. Also, if there is hot pink carpeting in the suite and you hate pink, the value of the carpeting is zero.

Accounts Receivable

Accounts receivable are the total amounts due directly from patients, insurance carriers, workers' compensation, and so on. The best way to get a value on accounts receivable is to "age" them, which involves going through all the accounts to determine how many are 30, 60, 90, 120, and over 180 days old. Assume that you will be able to collect only 50 percent of any accounts over 180 days old, 60 percent of those over 120 days, 80 percent of the accounts over 90 days, and 95 percent of those 30 days old or less. Usually, in a well-run practice, 95 to 98 percent of all gross billings are collectible. Accounts receivable are nothing more than payments due to the practice for services rendered.

Real Estate

The most precise way to value the building is to have it assessed by a professional appraiser, which will cost about $400 to $600. You can get an approximate estimate of the value by having a real estate agent determine the price he would set if he put the building on the market. For a very rough estimate, you could assume $60 per square foot, which is the current cost to build a new building.

Medical Records

The intangible value of medical records is increased if the physician is prepared to send a letter to the patients letting them know that the chart will be there and also will be in good hands. The value of the record per se is negligible; however, where the record resides is important.

Cash and Equivalents

Money in checking accounts, prepaid expenses, petty cash, stamp and postage meters, and comparable items are included in the category of cash and equivalents.

Valuing Intangible Assets

Valuing your tangible assets is relatively straightforward compared with setting a worth for the intangible aspects of the practice. However, it is the intangible assets (Figure 34-2) that allow a practice to be competitive, and they can increase the value of a practice tenfold. When one practice sells for a significantly higher price than another, it does so because of its intangible assets. These assets break down into three basic categories: (1) factors that will ensure continuing patient flow; (2) those that maximize financial stability; and (3) those that affect the quality of the practice and patient care. There are no absolute rules for placing a dollar value on these items. I have seen practices for sale that have valued intangibles at from $10,000 to as much as $60,000, with the average about $30,000.

Figure 34-2

Practice Valuation Work Sheet—Intangible Assets

---

1. **Factors that affect patient flow**   _____

   a   Significant demographic trends   _____

   b   Transferability of patients   _____

   c   "Interesting" practice   _____

   d   Source of referral   _____

   e   Location   _____

   f   Seller's willingness to assist in transfer   _____

   g   Employee retention   _____

   h   _____   _____

   i   _____   _____

2. **Factors that affect financial stability**   _____

   a   Gross receipts   _____

   b   Net income before taxes   _____

   c   Collection ratio   _____

   d   Fees   _____

   e   Size of patient roster   _____

   f   Telephone number   _____

   g   Practice name   _____

3. **Quality of patient care**   _____

   a   Quality of staff   _____

   b   Systems and procedures   _____

   c   Quality of usable space   _____

   d   Patient mix   _____

   e   Atmosphere   _____

4. **Miscellaneous considerations**   _____

   a   Specialty   _____

   b   Covenant not to compete   _____

   c   Reason for sale   _____

Total intangible assets   _____

Patient Flow

One pediatrician found that many of his patients had moved away and what was once an area with many children was now a quiet area with many happy grandparents. As a result, because of demographic factors, the practice was worth significantly less than that of the pediatrician who purchased a practice in a booming area where new families were having children.

Transferability of Patients

The value of the transferability of patients can be increased if the seller of the practice is prepared to stay on for a few months or be available as a consultant to the practice. Also, if the seller is prepared to leave his name on the practice for three years or so, this also increases the transferability of the patients. As part of the sales agreement, the departing physician should be prepared to send a letter to all the patients introducing the buyer.

"Interesting" Practice

A practice that has many interesting cases rather than just routine ones may be worth more for intrinsic reasons. For example, an ophthalmology practice with patients who are primarily surgical cases may be worth more than a practice that mainly involves refractions, because the practitioner is doing more complex and more highly skilled work.

Sources of Referral

How are referrals being generated in the practice? And, more important, would these referrals continue if a new person were to take over the practice? Perhaps more than any other intangible aspect, a good analysis of referral sources is critical. If the practice has a large and diverse referral base, this is far better than a few referral sources that account for the major part of the practice. If there are a small number of sources, the buyer will want to ensure that these sources will continue to refer patients to the practice. This may mean some specific discussions with the key referral sources before the purchase, in the case of a secondary care practice.

Location

Location has a tremendous bearing on the value of the practice. If patients have been coming to a particular location for the past 50 years for medical care because it is on an easily accessible corner with plenty of parking, the location is worth much more than a practice on an out-of-the-way street where people rarely travel.

Helpfulness of Seller

The seller's willingness to assist in the transfer of the practice provides greater selling power. In this situation the seller stays around for a minimum of three months to introduce the new physician to patients and referral sources, and he or she sends out letters to both groups introducing the new person. It is also of great help if the original physician can assist the new practitioner obtain hospital privileges and introduce him or her to community leaders.

Employees' Willingness to Stay

Continuity of practice is critical. Many times, although a physician is leaving, if a favorite nurse or receptionist remains this adds significant value to the practice. You might have the employee sign an employment contract for one or two years to ensure that he or she stays around with the new practitioner.

Financial Stability

Financial stability can be analyzed by looking at the last three years of gross receipts as well as net income before taxes. It is a good sign if practice net income has grown in that period. Examine the collection ratio—that is, how many accounts are actually being collected (total collections divided by gross billing); a 95 percent collection ratio is excellent. Anything less than 90 percent is questionable. The practice name is also valuable, especially if it is easily transferable or may be left listed in the yellow pages after you have left.

Quality of Practice/Patient Care

Staff members who are qualified, trained, and motivated increase practice value. It has been estimated that it can cost $1,000 to $2,000 to recruit a good quality staff member, and $5,000 to $10,000 to train one properly. As a result, there can be a large investment in experienced staff, an asset that is often overlooked. Efficient systems and procedures also increase the value of the practice since more patients can be seen with less cost in this type of practice.

Patient Mix

Patient mix should be considered. A practice with positive, happy patients who comply with your instructions is worth far more than one with transient patients whom you may see only once before they move on to another town and who have no insurance or insurance that pays poorly. It is also generally believed that a practice with most patients owning private insurance is worth more. Some final considerations are the specialty of the practice, the reason for the sale, and whether a convenant not to compete is included in the sale. The noncompetition covenant is often included because the person purchasing the practice from you wants to ensure that you cannot come back, set up a practice in the area, and recapture the patients who had been with you originally.

Figure 34-3

Practice Valuation Work Sheet—Liabilities

1. Mortgage   _____

2. Tax obligations   _____

3. Bank loans   _____

4. Insurance to be paid   _____

5. Unpaid bills   _____

6. Staff emoluments   _____

7. Damage under lease   _____

8. Impending lawsuits   _____

9. Other liabilities   _____

Total liabilities   _____

Practice value

(Tangible assets + Intangible assets − Liabilities) =   _____

Liabilities

The last step is to deduct all the liabilities (Figure 34-3) from the tangible and intangible assets. Liabilities include:

1. Mortgage outstanding
2. Tax obligations
3. Bank loans
4. Insurance to be paid
5. Staff emoluments
6. Unpaid bills
7. Potential damage under the lease
8. Impending lawsuits
9. Other liabilities

By totaling all these obligations and subtracting this amount from your assets, you will have a fair idea of the net worth of your practice. In other words, you will have completed your financial x-ray.

In a competitive era, the strategy of purchasing your practice has many benefits in the growth process. In business terms, this is called an acquisition. Large clinics will contemplate purchasing practices, as will new doctors starting up. Practice values will increase as competition intensifies. Your ability to assess and evaluate a practice's true potential can significantly aid your own growth and assist you in purchasing a practice or selling one—certainly valuable information to understand.

●

Chapter 35

The Business of Practicing Medicine

The art and science of practicing medicine is not a business, but there is a business involved in the peripheral aspects of ensuring that the service is delivered (that is, what I have termed *practice enhancement*). There is a fine distinction between delivering medical care and delivering the overall service to patients. Medical school does not train you to run a business, and you do not need to understand business principles to deliver care in its purest sense. However, there are a number of management aspects that must be attended to in a practice to ensure that the most effective level of care is delivered.

This chapter deals with business philosophy and its application to a practice enhancement program. As is true for operators of other small businesses, you will encounter many pressures in running your practice on a day-to-day basis that are not related to the actual medical care rendered. However, to deliver optimum medical care, you must ensure that all the business details are attended to. As in a small business, if your patients are unhappy and do not use your services, you become insolvent. In the new competitive era, more and more physicians will go bankrupt.

It is important for you to recognize that although you have been trained to be a doctor first, your next greatest responsibility is to the practice and the administrative details associated with the delivery of care. To succeed in the competitive era, you must be not only an excellent doctor but also an excellent business operator. Practice enhancement can bridge the gap.

Just as there are many complexities involved in the practice of medicine, so there are similar complexities in the administrative aspects of your practice. As in a small business, a medical practice must deal with all the traditional problems encountered by management—accounting and financial control, personnel administration, services delivery, and marketing. The emphasis on the problem relates to the era; currently, the emphasis is on marketing because of physician oversupply. By taking the best of what marketing has to offer, practice enhancement can help you bridge the gap.

Keeping Score for Practice Success

Perhaps one of the most common problems you face can be generally termed *keeping score,* or accounting and financial control. This topic, which was discussed earlier in the book, relates to the bookkeeping and management accounting procedures used to manage your cash flow; it includes billing, accounts receivable, accounts payable, and purchasing.

Figure 35-1 is an example of a cash flow form. As the person responsible for the practice, you should ensure that these systems are well implemented in your practice. You have to decide how to tackle the various business problems in the practice. You can put your head in the sand and rationalize that if you are a good doctor and provide good medical care the rest will take care of itself. I believe, however, that the successful practitioner in the competitive era will be successful because he or she is also a good business person and applies practice enhancement techniques. You need to begin with a plan to ensure that your practice enhancement plan is as sound as the treatment you provide to your patients.

As medicine becomes more competitive, it is more important than ever that your medical office be a well-run business. Operators of successful small businesses seek competent advice through business training to prepare themselves to meet their customer service and personal income objectives. Some standard solutions—such as budgeting, monthly management reports, time standards for systems and procedures, and marketing surveys—have been developed to aid

Figure 35-1. Sample of a cash flow chart.

	Jan.	Feb.	Mar.	Apr.	May	June	July	Aug.	Sept.	Oct.	Nov.	Dec.	Total
Income													
Total													
Expenditures													
Regular checks regular amounts													
Regular checks, varying amounts													
Irregular check payments													
Cash payments													
Total													
Overspent													
Underspent													
Total													
Expenditures													
Plus savings													
Savings account													
Balance (Dec.)													

265

in solving recurring business problems. Many of these business principles and techniques have proved to be extremely valuable when applied to meet the prime objective of a medical practice, which is to deliver the highest quality care at the lowest possible cost and to keep your patients satisfied.

When you set up and run your own medical practice you are running a small business. Your product is delivering high quality medical care to your patient/client at the lowest possible cost. Like the operator of any other small business, you have pressures in running your practice on a day-to-day basis that can be extensive since you must function in two roles. You deliver the service, but you also manage the business. You are independent and decisive, you work long hours, and each administrative decision you make ultimately affects your bottom-line income.

As in any small business, if your patients/clients are unhappy and do not use your services, you become insolvent or, more likely, you become what is called in business circles the "living dead"—someone whose business earns enough income to justify its continued existence but never realizes its ultimate service and income goals!

As a physician it is important for you to recognize that, although you are a healer first, your next greatest responsibility to your practice is administrative and it is for this reason that you are running a small business! To be successful in your practice you should follow the lead of successful small business operators who make it a policy to seek competent business advice and training for themselves. In that way you can prepare yourself to handle complex administrative problems as they affect your practice.

Cash Flow Problems

Did you ever realize that a one-week delay in processing your billings means that your practice has to provide financing, for that week, from some other source? In other words, if you pay your aides' salaries on the fifteenth of every month out of your medical insurance check (which usually arrives on or before that date) you have to meet those salaries on the fifteenth from another source if the insurance check is delayed. Many physicians and other operators of small businesses receive telephone calls from a bank manager in response to an overdrawn checking account—often the problem had previously not been noticed.

One general practitioner in Rochester can be used as an example of this type of problem, which was caused by inadequate planning of cash flow. Since his practice was growing, he was incurring additional costs in part-time salaries and general operating expenses. Furthermore, he was paying a number of lump sum irregular payments. Part of the problem stemmed from a recent purchase of substantially more life insurance without examining the cash flow pattern of his practice. On the income side, he was billing the medical plan substantially more but not receiving payment for his work until two or three months later. As a result, a cash flow imbalance developed that resulted in a call from his bank manager informing him of his somewhat large overdraft. After seeking advice, he instituted a monthly practice cash flow report that was prepared for the next 12 months (see Figure 35-1). A schedule of receipts from all sources was estimated, giving consideration to income resulting from practice growth. Regular and irregular payments were estimated and any additional planned expenditures were added.

The second step in the Rochester physician's reorganization was to train his aide to complete a report using the same format to reflect, in summary, what actually happened in the past month. In this way he could review his practice financial picture on a regular basis and make changes to his projected financial status as unexpected occurrences affected his practice. He later acknowledged that the report helped him to realize that he could increase his cash flow considerably by making sure all the billings went out daily. At first it seemed like an enormous task, but he found it relatively easy after the bugs in the billing system were eliminated.

Preparing a simple cash budget and sticking to that plan will simplify your life immensely in terms of planning your cash needs. In that way you can avoid the problems of the many physicians who are "paper rich but cash poor."

Personnel Problems

Personnel presents probably the second most common problem in small businesses, particularly in medical practices. Few doctors have not had a bad experience with the quality or volume of staff members' output. The staff in one physician's office was continually complaining that there was too much work to be done and that more people would be needed if all tasks were to be completed. In addition, staff turnover was high, accounts were not being billed regularly, and there was a general decline in the physician's patient roster. Furthermore, pressure was put on the physician for higher salaries. Therefore, personnel costs were rising as a percentage of other practice expenses. With some management assistance, a simple work measurement study was completed, detailing all of the office systems and procedures with time standards. It was estimated fewer people could handle a streamlined system to do all of the work. Detailed job definitions were written, including estimated standards for completing each clerical and paramedical task. After the reorganization, the office managed to complete all of the work with three people rather than four, and the doctor could then afford to raise salaries. The staff seemed happier because they had more direction, knowing exactly how and when each job should be completed.

Practice Location

A classic marketing problem encountered by all young physicians is where to locate their practice. This marketing function has been described by the American Management Association as "focusing your business on your customer's needs and desires, including those needs and desires the customer is not aware of and using this knowledge to ensure that your goods and/or services are bought." Therefore, in locating a medical practice it is important to understand both the stated and unstated needs and wishes of patients as they pertain to the selection of a new primary care physician. In the long run, a well-chosen location will serve as an effective promotional device for your practice. Therefore, an appropriate location for a new practice is a very important factor for long-term planning. In the event of problems in this area, however, business solutions are available.

One example of such solutions can be seen in two general practitioners who, after lengthy deliberation, established their practices in downtown Syracuse, N.Y. Although they originally perceived a need for additional medical service in the downtown area and were satisfied with convenient public transportation and reasonable rent, eight months later their practices were growing extremely slowly and both doctors were, in fact, in financial trouble.

After seeking advice, a market survey was conducted with the downtown population to get a better understanding of their needs and desires. Area merchants were interviewed regarding business trends. Some interesting facts were discovered:

1. Many of the merchants who had been doing well two years previously were then experiencing general declines in sales.
2. The reason for the decline was attributed to the trend of people toward suburban activity. Large plazas and shopping malls were

springing up. Old customers stopped going downtown as frequently.

3. By far the largest population in the downtown area were the office workers who commuted daily.

4. A significant need for additional medical services was found to exist only during the hours before and after work.

These physicians resolved their problems when one moved his practice to a small plaza that serviced a local community and the other changed his office hours to 7–9 A.M., 11–1 P.M., and 4–7 P.M. to accommodate the downtown office population. A year later the patient rosters of both practices were growing at a healthy rate. As you can see, when physicians are attuned to the real needs of the community, their practices prosper.

Business techniques developed for production planning in a small business can also be seen in another application, to the case of a busy pediatrician's practice in Buffalo:

1. The waiting room was either overcrowded or almost empty.

2. Patients and staff members were bumping into each other in the halls.

3. The nurses' station lacked privacy.

4. The business office was cramped and almost always untidy.

5. The practice was experiencing high staff turnover.

Solutions to these problems were found by applying the techniques of production planning, layout design, and scheduling. Patient flow and drop-in patterns were analyzed in detail. A work-flow study and a careful examination of space utilization led to changes in which some internal walls were eliminated and the nurses' station was enlarged by using one of the examining rooms for a dual purpose. Work units were constructed in the business office at low cost by a local carpenter. A flexible appointment system to control patient flow through the practice was implemented, and aides were trained to monitor the appointment system strictly.

Practice Is Small Business

Many doctors, including those described in this chapter, never thought of their practice as being a small business. However, as medicine becomes more competitive, it is more important than ever that your medical office be a well-run business. Successful small business operators seek competent advice and use business training to prepare themselves to meet their customer service and personal income objectives. Some standard solutions, such as budgeting, monthly summary management reporting, time standards for systems and procedures, and marketing surveys, have been developed to aid in solving recurring business problems. Many of these business principles and techniques have proved to be extremely valuable when applied to meet the prime objective of medical practice—which is to deliver the highest quality medical care at the lowest possible cost.

Bibliography

"Ads Start to Take Hold in the Professions." *Business Week,* July 24, 1978.

Block, Lee F. (ed.). *Marketing for Hospitals in Hard Times.* Chicago: Teach 'em, Inc., 1981.

Braun, Irwin. *Building A Successful Professional Practice with Advertising.* New York: Amacom, 1981.

Cooper, Philip D. *Health Care Marketing: Issues and Trends.* Orem, Utah: Aspen Publications, 1979.

Cooper, Philip D. (ed.). *Health Care Marketing.* Germantown, Md.: Aspen Systems, 1979.

Haver, Jurgen F. *Personalized Guide to Marketing Strategy.* St. Louis: Mosby, 1982.

Heiser, Ralph A. *Marketing Dental Services Professionally.* Edina, Minn.: Institute for Marketing Professional Services, 1981.

Kotler, Philip. *Marketing Management.* Englewood Cliffs, N.J.: Prentice-Hall, 1976.

Macstravic, Robin E. *Marketing Health Care.* Germantown, Md.: Aspen Systems, 1977.

Malickson, David L., and Nason, John W. *Advertising—How to Write the Works.* New York: Scribner's, 1977.

Milone, Charles L., Blair, Charles W., and Littlefield, James E. *Marketing for the Dental Practice.* Philadelphia: Saunders, 1982.

Rubright, Robert, and MacDonald, Dan. *Marketing Health and Human Services.* Rockville, Md.: Aspen Systems, 1981.

Smith, Cynthia S. *How to Get Big Results From a Small Advertising Budget.* New York: Hawthorn, 1973.

Snyder, Thomas L. *Personalized Guide to Practice Evaluation.* St. Louis, Mosby, 1982.

Walker, Morton. *Advertising and Promoting the Professional Practice.* New York: Hawthorn, 1979.

Weiner, Richard. *Professional's Guide to Public Relations Services* (3rd ed.). New York: Richard Weiner, Inc., 1975.

Wilson, Aubrey. *The Marketing of Professional Services.* New York: McGraw-Hill, 1972.

Index